The Ghrelin System

Endocrine Development

Vol. 25

Series Editor

P.-E. Mullis Bern

The Ghrelin System

Volume Editors

A. Benso Turin
F.F. Casanueva Santiago de Compostela
E. Ghigo Turin
R. Granata Turin

16 figures, 2 in color, and 4 tables, 2013

KARGER

Basel · Freiburg · Paris · London · New York · New Delhi · Bangkok · Beijing · Tokyo · Kuala Lumpur · Singapore · Sydney

Endocrine Development

Founded 1999 by Martin O. Savage, London

Andrea Benso
Division of Endocrinology, Diabetology and Metabolism
Department of Medical Sciences
University of Turin
Città della Salute e della Scienza University Hospital
Turin, Italy

Ezio Ghigo
Division of Endocrinology, Diabetology and Metabolism
Department of Medical Sciences
University of Turin
Città della Salute e della Scienza University Hospital
Turin, Italy

Felipe F. Casanueva
Laboratorio de Endocrinología Molecular nº 2,
Instituto de Investigaciones Sanitarias de Santiago de Compostela, Planta-2.
Complexo Hospitalario Universitario de Santiago
Santiago de Compostela, Spain

Riccarda Granata
Division of Endocrinology, Diabetology and Metabolism
Department of Medical Sciences
University of Turin
Città della Salute e della Scienza University Hospital
Turin, Italy

Library of Congress Cataloging-in-Publication Data

The ghrelin system / volume editors, A. Benso ... [et al.].
p. ; cm. -- (Endocrine development, ISSN 1421-7082 ; v. 25)
Includes bibliographical references and indexes.
ISBN 978-3-8055-9908-5 (hard cover : alk. paper) -- ISBN 978-3-8055-9909-2 (e-ISBN)
I. Benso, Andrea. II. Series: Endocrine development ; v. 25. 1421-7082
[DNLM: 1. Ghrelin--physiology. 2. Ghrelin--therapeutic use. W1 EN3635 v.25 2013 / WK 185]
RM286
615.3'6--dc23
2013009732

Bibliographic Indices. This publication is listed in bibliographic services, including Current Contents®.

Disclaimer. The statements, opinions and data contained in this publication are solely those of the individual authors and contributors and not of the publisher and the editor(s). The appearance of advertisements in the book is not a warranty, endorsement, or approval of the products or services advertised or of their effectiveness, quality or safety. The publisher and the editor(s) disclaim responsibility for any injury to persons or property resulting from any ideas, methods, instructions or products referred to in the content or advertisements.

Drug Dosage. The authors and the publisher have exerted every effort to ensure that drug selection and dosage set forth in this text are in accord with current recommendations and practice at the time of publication. However, in view of ongoing research, changes in government regulations, and the constant flow of information relating to drug therapy and drug reactions, the reader is urged to check the package insert for each drug for any change in indications and dosage and for added warnings and precautions. This is particularly important when the recommended agent is a new and/or infrequently employed drug.

www.karger.com
Printed in Germany on acid-free and non-aging paper (ISO 97069) by Kraft Druck GmbH, Ettlingen
ISSN 1421–7082
e-ISSN 1662–2979
ISBN 978–3–8055–9908–5
e-ISBN 978–3–8055–9909–2

Contents

Preface

It is our pleasure to welcome the reader to this book dedicated to ghrelin, a gastric hormone discovered in 1999 as the natural GH secretagogue that binds and activates the GHS receptor due to its particular mode of octanoylation in Ser3.

The ghrelin story is a story of reverse pharmacology which started more than 30 years ago with the discovery of synthetic non-natural growth hormone-releasing peptides. The following milestones of the story were the discovery of nonpeptidyl GHS and that of the GHS receptor. Following ghrelin's discovery, another major milestone has been the discovery of the specific acyltransferase (GOAT) able to acylate the peptide.

For many years, the ghrelin story was closely related to the regulation of GH secretion. We soon learnt that its action was not at all specific either from the endocrine or from the nonendocrine point of view. In the last decade, ghrelin became more famous as an orexigenic agent playing a major role in the control of food intake and energy expenditure. Research in this field has really provided new understanding in both neuroscience and metabolism. The last 10 years has also made it clear that ghrelin is much more than just a natural orexigenic factor. Besides other important central activities, it is now clear that ghrelin exerts major peripheral endocrine and nonendocrine actions. In particular, there is increasing evidence showing that ghrelin plays a key role in glucose metabolism and that it could have many clinical implications.

Final understanding of the physiological and pathophysiological roles of ghrelin is still awaited. However, a key concept we have already learnt is that ghrelin is an active peptide exerting remarkable metabolic actions even when it is not acylated. This implies a profound revision of the former vision as well as seeking out new perspectives for research and potential clinical indications.

Considering that this hormone is considered to play a relevant central role and that its peripheral actions include influence on behavior, hypothalamus-pituitary function, activity and secretion of peripheral endocrine glands, metabolic balance, gastroenteropancreatic function, cardiovascular function, and normal and neoplastic cell proliferation, it is now clear that the discovery of ghrelin was not just a milestone in neuroendocrinology but probably in medicine too.

We are indebted to all of the authors who contributed chapters for this book. Herein, you can find works by almost all of the scientists who have provided major contributions to this fascinating field.

It is our hope that this book will give readers an exhaustive picture of the present knowledge in the field of ghrelin research.

Given the impressive speed in the growing body of information and discoveries, it is clear that this book will soon be obsolete but nevertheless remain a good basis for a better understanding of the novelties awaiting us in the near future.

Andrea Benso, Turin
Felipe F. Casanueva, Santiago de Compostela
Ezio Ghigo, Turin
Riccarda Granata, Turin

Benso A, Casanueva FF, Ghigo E, Granata A (eds): The Ghrelin System.
Endocr Dev. Basel, Karger, 2013, vol 25, pp 1–4 (DOI: 10.1159/000346036)

Ghrelin Discovery: A Decade After

Masayasu Kojima[a] · Kenji Kangawa[b]

[a]Molecular Genetics, Institute of Life Science, Kurume University, Kurume, and
[b]National Cerebral and Cardiovascular Center Research Institute, Osaka, Japan

Abstract

Since its discovery 12 years ago, intensive research has been performed on ghrelin. The significance of ghrelin as a growth hormone-releasing hormone, appetite regulator, energy conservator and sympathetic nerve suppressor has now been well established. In this short essay, we summarize the history of the discovery of ghrelin.

Beginning

Everything has a beginning and an end. Sometimes a research ends with good results and sometimes it ends up as a failure. In the case of our ghrelin research, it ended with good results. If one of our team members, Kenji Kangawa, Hiroshi Hosoda, or I were not involved, ghrelin would not have been discovered. This short essay is a record of our research on ghrelin.

Our research style is 'in the beginning there was a novel peptide'. We have been searching for novel unknown peptides for almost 30 years. We discovered the opioid peptides (α-neoendorphin, etc.), neuromedins and the natriuretic peptide family (ANP, BNP and CNP). It is very exciting to find a novel peptide and explore unknown physiological functions. It is just like a treasure hunt or climbing a virgin peak.

Kenji and I moved from Miyazaki Medical College to the National Cardiovascular Center Research Institute in Osaka in 1993 and began to search for novel peptide hormones. However, we could not find any novel peptides for the first 6 years, except for known peptides and fragments derived from nonpeptide hormone proteins. Hiroshi joined us as a graduate student to take a PhD degree just before we had tackled the search for the endogenous ligand to the GHS-R.

From the beginning of 1998, we had been searching for the endogenous ligands of several orphan GPCRs, such as GHS-R, BRS-3, GPR37, GPR39, mas, etc., although none of the ligands except for ghrelin have yet been discovered. Among several of the orphan GPCRs that we searched, GHS-R (growth hormone secretagogue receptor) is somehow an exception [1]. Most of these orphan receptors did not have a specific activator; however, GHS-R had its specific activator GHSs, a group of synthetic compounds that stimulate GH release [2]. This means that the GHS-R assay system can be monitored.

Stomach

By January 1999, almost 1 year after we had started the ligand search for the GHS-R, we had found several peptides that activated the GHS-R; however, these peptides were always protein fragments, such as Purkinje cell protein 2 or myelin basic protein, and their activities were very low, indicating that these peptide fragments were not the real ligand for the GHS-R. We had undertaken many steps of chromatography and ran more than 500 assays and still had no hint of the ligand. We began to think that we should change the target from brain to other tissues.

At that time another orphan GPCR, GPR38, that shows high homology to GHS-R had already been known [3]. GPR38 was later identified as the motilin receptor [4]. In total deadlock, we began to think that because GHS-R and GPR38 have similar amino acid structures, their endogenous ligands should cross-react to the other receptor. Then, if we can find the GPR38 ligand, we can get some hint for the GHS-R ligand. Since GPR38 is highly expressed in the stomach and thyroid tissues, we began to assay GHS-R-expressing cells by using stomach extract. After the success of finding our ghrelin, we found that only our group had changed the target tissue and no other groups had tried stomach samples. This was very lucky for us, because content of ghrelin in the stomach was too high that every group should have succeeded to find the ligand, if only they tried to find it in the stomach.

A Novel Peptide

Unexpectedly, too high amounts of the endogenous ligand exist in the stomach. Several milligrams of the stomach extract is sufficient for detecting the activity. We only needed 10 days to complete the purification from 1 g of rat stomach tissue. However, amino acid sequence analysis of the purified ligand had given no signal at the third amino acid. From the cDNA analysis of the ligand, the unknown third amino acid was identified as a serine. We synthesized the ligand peptide and checked the activity, but there was none. We compared the purified and synthetic ligands and found that their elution positions on HPLC are very different, indicating that they have a different structure. One possibility is that the serine residue at the third position is modified by an unknown molecule and this modification should be necessary for the activity.

What is the modification? From the data of the molecular weight of the purified peptide, we speculated that modification of structure of the third serine to be with n-octanoic acid. Mixture of the natural and synthetic n-octanoyl peptides gave a single peak on HPLC, which means that the two peptides had a perfectly matched elution time. Then, we checked the GHS receptor-expressing cells to see whether the synthetic peptide had activated the cells. The activity of the synthetic peptide on the GHS receptor matched that of the natural peptide. Moreover, the synthetic and natural peptides showed the same profiles by their physical and chemical characters. Finally, we identified the structure as an acyl-modified peptide from the stomach [5]. We named this peptide 'ghrelin' derived from 'ghre', which means 'grow' in Indo-European roots. To our joy, the name is accepted by the research world.

After the Discovery of Ghrelin

After the discovery of ghrelin, we and other groups examined the physiological functions of ghrelin and found that ghrelin is a potent orexigenic hormone [6–8]. This was very exciting since ghrelin is a circulating hormone and these results indicated a future application of ghrelin for the treatment of eating disorders.

Another interesting point on ghrelin was the identification of the enzyme, ghrelin *O*-acyltransferase (GOAT), which modified and activated ghrelin. We had searched for the enzyme since the discovery of ghrelin. However, in 2008 two other groups reported the enzyme and we lost [9, 10]. The results were very surprising and exciting, because the enzyme was exclusively specific for the acyl modification of ghrelin. Thus, several inhibitors for GOAT may be useful for the treatment of metabolic disorders [11].

Moreover, it remained to be answered whether ghrelin is the only acyl-modified peptide hormone or not, because several orphan acyltransferases whose substrates have not yet been identified are registered in the genome database [12].

Recent developments in research technology enable us to challenge difficult questions in ghrelin research. For example, the crystal structure of the ghrelin receptor and 3-D analysis of the receptor activation will be characterized in the near future. How does the n-octanoyl moiety of ghrelin bind to the ghrelin receptor and why is the acyl modification necessary for receptor activation? These questions will be answered by the latest methods for determining the crystal structures of membrane proteins.

Epilogue

The discovery of ghrelin changed our (Kojima, Hiroshi and Kenji) lives, of course to a better one. However, even in these days I often imagine what would have happened in my research life if I had not changed the target tissue from brain to stomach or if I could not have solved the modified structure of ghrelin. We need some luck to get through to a good research. Although it may be a hackneyed phrase that whether you can get lucky or not depends on your passion for your research, I believe it.

Lastly, please let me express my personal pleasure. I am very very happy and honored to find that 'ghrelin' is described in *Lehninger's Biochemistry* and *Stryer's Biochemistry*, textbooks that I used for study in biochemical courses in my college student days. I could not have imagined when I was a young student that a discovery of mine would be in these textbooks 30 years later.

References

1 Howard AD, Feighner SD, Cully DF, Arena JP, Liberator PA, Rosenblum CI, Hamelin M, Hreniuk DL, Palyha OC, Anderson J, Paress PS, Diaz C, Chou M, Liu KK, McKee KK, Pong SS, Chaung LY, Elbrecht A, Dashkevicz M, Heavens R, Rigby M, Sirinathsinghji DJ, Dean DC, Melillo DG, Patchett AA, Nargund R, Griffin PR, DeMartino JA, Gupta SK, Schaeffer JM, Smith RG, Van der Ploeg LH: A receptor in pituitary and hypothalamus that functions in growth hormone release. Science 1996;273:974–977.

2 Bowers CY: Growth hormone-releasing peptide (GHRP). Cell Mol Life Sci 1998;54:1316–1329.

3 McKee KK, Tan CP, Palyha OC, Liu J, Feighner SD, Hreniuk DL, Smith RG, Howard AD, Van der Ploeg LH: Cloning and characterization of two human G protein-coupled receptor genes (GPR38 and GPR39) related to the growth hormone secretagogue and neurotensin receptors. Genomics 1997;46:426–434.

4 Feighner SD, Tan CP, McKee KK, Palyha OC, Hreniuk DL, Pong SS, Austin CP, Figueroa D, MacNeil D, Cascieri MA, Nargund R, Bakshi R, Abramovitz M, Stocco R, Kargman S, O'Neill G, Van Der Ploeg LH, Evans J, Patchett AA, Smith RG, Howard AD: Receptor for motilin identified in the human gastrointestinal system. Science 1999;284:2184–2188.

5 Kojima M, Hosoda H, Date Y, Nakazato M, Matsuo H, Kangawa K: Ghrelin is a growth-hormone-releasing acylated peptide from stomach. Nature 1999;402: 656–660.

6 Nakazato M, Murakami N, Date Y, Kojima M, Matsuo H, Kangawa K, Matsukura S: A role for ghrelin in the central regulation of feeding. Nature 2001;409: 194–198.

7 Tschop M, Smiley DL, Heiman ML: Ghrelin induces adiposity in rodents. Nature 2000;407:908–913.

8 Wren AM, Small CJ, Ward HL, Murphy KG, Dakin CL, Taheri S, Kennedy AR, Roberts GH, Morgan DG, Ghatei MA, Bloom SR: The novel hypothalamic peptide ghrelin stimulates food intake and growth hormone secretion. Endocrinology 2000;141:4325–4328.

9 Gutierrez JA, Solenberg PJ, Perkins DR, Willency JA, Knierman MD, Jin Z, Witcher DR, Luo S, Onyia JE, Hale JE: Ghrelin octanoylation mediated by an orphan lipid transferase. Proc Natl Acad Sci USA 2008; 105:6320–6325.

10 Yang J, Brown MS, Liang G, Grishin NV, Goldstein JL: Identification of the acyltransferase that octanoylates ghrelin, an appetite-stimulating peptide hormone. Cell 2008;132:387–396.

11 Barnett BP, Hwang Y, Taylor MS, Kirchner H, Pfluger PT, Bernard V, Lin YY, Bowers EM, Mukherjee C, Song WJ, Longo PA, Leahy DJ, Hussain MA, Tschop MH, Boeke JD, Cole PA: Glucose and weight control in mice with a designed ghrelin *O*-acyltransferase inhibitor. Science 2010;330:1689–1692.

12 Hofmann K: A superfamily of membrane-bound *O*-acyltransferases with implications for wnt signaling. Trends Biochem Sci 2000;25:111–112.

Masayasu Kojima
Molecular Genetics, Institute of Life Science
Kurume-University
Kurume, Fukuoka 839-0864 (Japan)
E-Mail kojima_masayasu@kurume-u.ac.jp

Benso A, Casanueva FF, Ghigo E, Granata A (eds): The Ghrelin System.
Endocr Dev. Basel, Karger, 2013, vol 25, pp 5–15 (DOI: 10.1159/000346042)

The Ghrelin Receptors (GHS-R1a and GHS-R1b)

Rosie G. Albarrán-Zeckler · Roy G. Smith

Smith Laboratory, Department of Metabolism and Aging, The Scripps Research Institute, Scripps Florida, Jupiter, Fla., USA

Abstract

The growth hormone (GH) secretagogue receptor (GHS-R1a) is a G protein-coupled receptor (GPCR) expressed in the brain as well as other areas of the body. In the early 1990s, this receptor was expression cloned in MERCK laboratories by using a group of synthesized small molecules known to increase GH release in humans and other animals. Since its discovery, hundreds of studies have shown the importance of this receptor and its endogenous ligand, ghrelin, in metabolism, neurotransmission, and behavior. Even more relevant are the prospective benefits that will result from pharmacologic manipulation of GHS-R1a. Multiple GHS-R1a agonists and antagonists are available for experimentation, and some have been used in patients with promising results. Studies in rodents have revealed intriguing potential roles for GHS-R1a modulation. Our goal in this chapter is to connect these studies with the inherent advantages of targeting this receptor pharmacologically.

Ghrelin activation of the ghrelin receptor, GHS-R1a, has many regulatory effects on physiology and behavior, such as enhancement of memory and learning, neuroprotection, immune function improvement, blood glucose control, potentiation of drug and food addiction, and cardiovascular and renal protection [1–9]. Based on the results of these studies, in this chapter we will explore the potential benefits of pharmacological regulation of the GHS-R1a in disease states and aging. Furthermore, during the last decade, our laboratory has pioneered studies showing that the GHS-R1a heterodimerizes with other G protein-coupled receptors (GPCRs), such as the dopamine receptor type 1 (D1R) and type 2 (D2R), and that these interactions influence their signaling pathways [10, 11]. Based on our observations, we hypothesize that many of the reported in vivo results between the dopaminergic and ghrelin systems are most likely due to the physical interactions of these receptors. In addition, we have observed in our laboratory that the GHS-R1a knockout (*ghsr–/–*) mouse is refractory to the anorexigenic effects D2R agonists. Since these heterodimers exist in specific subsets of neurons [11], we postulate that molecules specifically targeting these heterodimers would potentially alleviate certain conditions, with the advantage of having fewer side effects. Indeed, during the last decade, multiple studies have reported the existence of GPCRs heterodimers, and it is believed that finding drugs that target these heterodimers alone will improve treatment specificity [12].

History

The amplitude of growth hormone (GH) release is gradually reduced with age, which results in a progressive health decline. GH replacement is not a satisfactory treatment because it can only be delivered by injection, which results in a one-time high-dose peak, instead of the periodic pulses naturally observed in humans in a 24-hour period. Therefore, in the early 1990s, a group of scientists at Merck laboratories were interested in finding a suitable molecule, with high oral bioavailability, that would stimulate the natural episodic release of GH [13, 14]. At that time, it had been reported that a small peptide composed of 6 amino acid residues, GHRP-6, had GH-releasing actions both in vitro and in vivo [15]; however, its mechanism of action was unknown. The Merck group initiated a series of studies in primary cultures of rat pituitary cells to elucidate the mechanism of action of GHRP-6. The results of these studies showed that GHRP-6 acted on a receptor distinct from that of the GH-releasing hormone (GHRH) receptor and somatostatin receptors. In addition to inducing GH release from pituicytes, GHRP-6 augmented both GHRH-induced cAMP accumulation and GH release. It was also shown to be a functional antagonist of somatostatin. Based on these properties and the chemical structure of GHRP-6, a chemical library was screened to identify nonpeptide mimetics. Subsequently, a series of nonpeptide mimetics (MK0677, L-692,429), with potent GH-stimulating properties, were developed [13, 14, 16]. Interestingly, and in accordance with previous reports on GHRP-6, MK0677 and L-692,429 appeared to activate a receptor not yet described in the literature. Evidence for a new receptor included that both GHRP-6 and MK0677 were able to stimulate GH release in the presence of a GHRH-R antagonist [17], and that a potentiation of GH release was observed when GHRH and MK0677 were given together, compared to each alone. Besides their action on pituitary cells, GHRP-6 and its mimetics activated GHRH neurons in the arcuate nucleus of the hypothalamus [18].

Additional characterization revealed that MK0677 activated a calcium-dependent pathway, instead of the cAMP-dependent signaling observed upon activation of GHRH-R. This finding was crucial in the cloning of the new receptor because it allowed them to use aequorin, a protein known to liberate light upon calcium binding. By coexpressing aequorin, the G protein $G_{\alpha q11}$, and a polyA RNA library made from swine somatotrophs in *Xenopus* oocytes, clones containing the potential receptor were sequentially identified by measuring aequorin-dependent bioluminescence in response to MK0677 [17]. The coexpression of $G_{\alpha q11}$ was essential for reproducibly detecting MK0677 activation of Ca^{2+} in *Xenopus* oocytes because this G protein is required for calcium release from intracellular stores [17]. Two sequences were identified with this approach, and one of the sequences was a truncated version of the other. The encoded proteins revealed a seven transmembrane domain receptor, GHS-R1a, and a second nonfunctional receptor, GHS-R1b, containing only five transmembrane domains. Both, GHS-R1a and GHS-R1b, are encoded by the same gene located on chromosome 3q26.31 [19]. The GHS-R1a is conserved among many species, including rat, mouse, chicken, pufferfish and zebrafish [17], which is important because most studies that look at the actions of GHS-R1a are performed in rodents.

The endogenous ligand for this receptor, ghrelin, was identified by studying the activation of the GHS-R1a in the presence of extracts from various organs [20]. It was found by Kojima et al. [20] that ghrelin is synthesized and released from the stomach and travels through the bloodstream to activate the ghrelin receptor expressed in other areas of the body such as the pancreas, hypothalamus, thymus and heart. Ghrelin is made in its inactive form, un-acylated or des-acyl ghrelin, but acylation of the third serine by ghrelin *O*-acyltransferase (GOAT) is subsequently required for ghrelin's activation of the GHS-R1a [19, 21–23]. Actions of des-acyl ghrelin are beyond the scope of this chapter because the GHS-R1a is not activated by the un-acylated form of ghrelin.

Following ghrelin's discovery, it was established that this hormone stimulates appetite by activating presynaptic GHS-R1a located in neuronal projections from the lateral hypothalamus, and stimulating the release of orexigenic hormones, such as neuropeptide Y (NPY) and Agouti-related peptide (AgRP) into the paraventricular nucleus, an area of the hypothalamus known to control food intake and appetite [24, 25]. Ghrelin binding initiates coupling of GHSR-1a to the heterotrimeric G protein $G_{\alpha q11}$, which activates a phospholipase C-dependent pathway and induces intracellular calcium mobilization from endoplasmic reticulum (ER) stores. Although ghrelin is mainly known for these orexigenic actions, the broad expression of the GHS-R1a in the body is indicative of its other regulatory effects.

The GHS-R1b is a splice variant and a dominant negative form of GHS-R1a [26]. Leung et al. [26] have almost exclusively studied GHS-R1b regulatory action, in comparison to GHS-R1a. Their data suggest that GHS-R1b heterodimerizes with GHS-R1a in HEK 293 cells, as shown by bioluminescence resonance energy transfer experiments. They further found that such heterodimerization decreases [^{125}I]ghrelin binding at the plasma membrane when GHS-R1b, which is not capable of binding ghrelin, was expressed at least 5 times more than GHS-R1a [26]. Imaging with GFP-tagged GHS-R1a showed co-localization with markers for the plasma membrane, Golgi, and ER [27], whereas GFP-tagged GHS-R1b was only expressed in the ER. When GFP-tagged GHS-R1a was co-expressed with nontagged GHS-R1b, a decrease in GHS-R1a-GFP levels at the plasma membrane and Golgi was observed;

however, levels in the ER appeared unchanged [27]. Thus, it was proposed that GHS-R1b prevents GHS-R1a from leaving the ER and regulates its concentration on the plasma membrane [27]. Interestingly, coexpression of both receptors affects GHS-R1a dependent calcium signaling, but not ghrelin-induced ERK 1/2 phosphorylation [27].

GHS-R1a, Glucose Homeostasis and Obesity

Many have pointed to high levels of ghrelin as the culprit of obesity because ghrelin injections acutely increase food intake in rodents [24] and promote feelings of hunger in humans [28]. Paradoxically, ghrelin levels decrease with obesity and gradually increase with weight loss [29, 30], and MK0677 increased lean mass in both elderly and obese patients with little effect on fat mass [31, 32]. Furthermore, *ghsr–/–* mice ingest similar quantities of chow and are relatively similar in weight and size to wild-type mice [33, 34], showing that GHS-R1a deletion does not alter feeding patterns. Mice lacking the appetite suppressing hormone leptin *(ob/ob)* are grossly overweight and present high levels of blood glucose, resembling type 2 diabetes [35, 36], and it was hypothesized that deletion of ghrelin would improve their condition. Unexpectedly, it was demonstrated that mice lacking both ghrelin and leptin (*ghrelin–/–* × *ob/ob*) were not leaner than the *ob/ob* mice, but had improved glucose clearance and increased insulin sensitivity [25, 35]. These data collectively argue that ghrelin is unlikely a sole cause of obesity, and instead just one component of a complex network regulating food intake and energy expenditure. Nevertheless, this work does suggest that GHS-R1a antagonism may improve hyperglycemia in humans.

GHS-R1a in the Brain

In the brain, the GHS-R1a is expressed in the hippocampus, the ventral tegmental area (VTA), substantia nigra (SN), and dorsal raphe nucleus [6, 25]. These areas are important for cognition, reward, motor control, and anxiety, respectively. To date, there is no convincing evidence that ghrelin is made in the brain [37]. In most of the in vivo studies in which ghrelin was shown to increase memory and learning or dopamine neurotransmission, ghrelin was delivered either intracerebroventricularly or via minipumps, which could lead to extremely high circulating ghrelin concentrations [1]. However, the broad expression of the GHS-R1a in the brain allows for pharmacological manipulation and potential treatments for various diseases such as Alzheimer's disease, Parkinson's disease, schizophrenia, posttraumatic stress disorder, and age-related memory loss. The following subsections explain how GHS-R1a expression modulates signaling of other neurotransmitters, as well as the benefits of GHS-R1a agonism during aging and other diseases.

GHS-R1a Heterodimerization with Dopamine Receptors in the Brain

Fluorescence resonance energy transfer and bioluminescence resonance energy transfer technologies have been crucial to discovery of GPCR heterodimers. Examples of dimers and higher order oligomers between different families of GPCRs exist throughout the literature [12, 38]. The GHS-R1a was shown to dimerize with the D1R [10] and D2R [11] and with the melanocortin receptor type 3 (MC3R) [39]. Formation of these dimers dramatically influences the signaling of the receptors. In vitro, ghrelin acts through the GHS-R1a to potentiate D1R-induced cAMP accumulation [10], and coincidentally GHS-R1a also augments MC3R-induced cAMP levels [39]. In addition, GHS-R1a coexpression with D2R in HEK 293 cells results in dopamine-induced intracellular calcium mobilization, which does not occur in the same cells expressing D2R alone [11]. It is important to stress that ghrelin was not present in the D2R studies, suggesting that in the brain, the GHS-R1a can modulate cellular signaling and behavior even in the absence of ghrelin. These data also provide further evidence that the GHS-R1a can regulate neurotransmission in the brain.

In vivo, our results show that the GHS-R1a is required for dopamine-regulated behavior [7, 11]. Dopamine neurotransmission into the nucleus accumbens is required for exploratory behaviors and motivation. In addition, when D1R signaling was blocked in the hippocampus, rats were less able to remember aversive stimuli in a step down test [40], indicating that dopamine signaling through this receptor is also important for memory acquisition. In our studies, *ghsr–/–* mice were less active after adaptation to a novel environment and showed impaired contextual memory in the fear conditioning paradigm, which measures the ability to remember an environment paired with an aversive stimulus (i.e. foot shock) [7]. Therefore, we conclude that dopamine signaling in these behaviors is regulated by GHS-R1a expression; ongoing experiments are exploring the relationship between D1R and GHS-R1a in vivo.

The D2R is expressed in hypothalamic neurons in the arcuate nucleus and activation of this receptor suppresses appetite. Interestingly, the D2R agonist cabergoline decreases food intake in wild-type and *ghrelin–/–* mice, but not *ghsr–/–* mice [11]. These findings suggest that GHSR-1a is required for dopamine mediated appetite suppression. Based on the heterodimerization results, it has been hypothesized that dopamine exerts its anorexic actions through activation of D2R/GHS-R1a heterodimers in the hypothalamus, independent of ghrelin.

Exogenous ghrelin, through GHS-R1a activation, enhances memory and learning in rodents [1]. Ghrelin also induces dopamine neurotransmission in rodents [6, 9, 41, 42], resulting in increased addictive behavior to both food and drugs of abuse, like alcohol and cocaine. Indeed, the GHS-R1a antagonist, JMV2959, prevented cocaine-induced sensitization in the open field, which measures locomotor activity [43]. These studies show the importance of ghrelin in the brain, while also highlighting the potential therapeutic actions of GHS-R1a regulation using both agonists and antagonists. While GHS-R1a agonism could enhance cognition; antagonists could help in treatment of addiction or mental diseases where dopamine is overproduced, such as schizophrenia.

GHS-R1a and Neuroprotection

Accumulation of reactive oxygen species (ROS) increases with age, and is believed to be linked to neurodegenerative diseases such as Parkinson's disease, Alzheimer's disease, and dementia [44, 45]. Studies in mice where the ghrelin gene has been deleted (*ghrelin–/–*) highlight the ability of ghrelin signaling, through the GHS-R1a, to protect midbrain dopaminergic neurons against the toxin 1-methyl-4-phenyl-1,2,3,6-tetrahydropyridine, which models Parkinson's disease in rodents by increasing ROS [3, 46, 47]. Uncoupling protein 2 (UCP2) is expressed in the brain, and prevents ROS overproduction and accumulation by capturing protons (H^+) and returning them to the mitochondrial matrix [48]. Ghrelin is believed to induce fatty acid oxidation and, interestingly, Andrews et al. [3] found that mice lacking UCP2 (*ucp2–/–*) were more susceptible to ghrelin-induced oxidation compared to wild-type mice. In this study, ghrelin was not able to protect against 1-methyl-4-phenyl-1,2,3,6-tetrahydropyridine insults in *ucp2–/–* mice, but was effective in their wild-type equivalents [3]. More recently, ghrelin was shown to protect primary neurons from ER stress [49]. Thus, GHS-R1a agonists could potentially be used to prevent aging-related and/or environmental-induced ROS production and accumulation.

Impact of GHS-R1a Activation in the Cardiovascular System

GHS-R1a expression has also been observed in the heart ventricles and atria, pulmonary artery, coronary artery, and aorta in rodents and humans [28, 30, 50, 51]. Nagaya et al. [28] were the first group to study the benefits of ghrelin in the cardiovascular system in healthy patients. They found that intravenous ghrelin improved total stroke volume coming from the left ventricle (cardiac output) and lowered blood pressure without affecting heart rate [28]. In a subsequent study, subcutaneous ghrelin injections also increased cardiac output in healthy 30-year-old males, as observed by decreased blood volume inside the left ventricle after systole [51].

Since ghrelin and other GHSR-1a agonists are protective against ischemia-induced heart failure in rats [52–54] and inflammation in human artery cells [50], it has been proposed that ghrelin or GHS-R1a agonists treatment could potentially improve blood flow and heart function in cases of arteriosclerosis, diabetes, and other heart diseases in humans. Promising results were obtained in patients suffering from myocardial infarction (heart attack); ghrelin treatment for 3 weeks showed better cardiac output and improved capacity under physical activity, as observed by increased oxygen consumption [55].

The ghrelin delivery method has proven to be important as well. For example, when ghrelin was given subcutaneously, blood pressure and the stress hormone, cortisol, were unaffected [51]; whereas intravenous ghrelin elevated cortisol and reduced blood pressure [28]. Acute subcutaneous ghrelin increased GH blood levels for 1–2 h after treatment, indicating that this method is sufficient to reach results similar to the obtained by intravenous ghrelin injections (the peaks of cortisol and GH occur simultaneously within minutes – they probably did not look at these early time points) [51]. Since GH also has positive effects on cardiovascular health, ghrelin's actions are twofold: it directly activates GHS-R1a in heart and artery cells and indirectly triggers GH release [28].

Although these results show a beneficial effect of acute ghrelin treatment, as discussed above, ghrelin injections are not a good replacement therapy because it has to be administered by injection and has a very short half-life. Thus, long-term studies with orally bioavailable GHS-R1a agonists with extended half-lives that improve episodic GH release are necessary in order to determine the efficacy of this treatment in chronic heart conditions and blood flow. Such treatment may also prove beneficial for cognition, since a decrease in blood flow, and thus oxygen, in the brain results in neuron death and memory deficits.

Potential Benefits of GHS-R1a Activation during Malnutrition and Cachexia

The prognosis for heart failure recovery declines when patients develop cachexia, which is a loss of lean body mass resulting from lack of appetite and malnutrition during serious illnesses [53]. Cachexia is also observed in cancer patients and those suffering from renal failure. Finding treatments that can improve nutrition, absorption, and body composition during chronic disease states like these is necessary. Studies in patients afflicted with either heart failure or cancer show elevated levels of ghrelin, but only in those simultaneously experiencing cachexia, suggesting that the human body has a restorative mechanism to increase ghrelin levels during undernourishment conditions [56, 57]. Studies using ghrelin and the peptide ghrelin mimetics BIM 28125 and BIM 28131 improved muscle strength and pain sensation and increased food intake and body weight gain in rats suffering from ischemic-induced heart failure or cisplatin-induced cachexia [53, 58]. Therefore, Garcia et al. [8] tested the effects of an oral ghrelin mimetic, anamorelin, in patients with cancer cachexia. In this study, anamorelin increased appetite, food intake, and GH levels, and improved overall mood in cachectic patients to levels present in healthy controls and cancer patients without cachexia [8]. While some patients reported nausea and high blood sugar, it was generally well tolerated. Clinical studies are continuing for the use of anamorelin in cancer cachexia patients and awaiting approval by the Food and Drug Administration in the United States.

GHS-R1a in Other Aging-Related Conditions

Thymocytes are crucial for the production of T cells, and thus the ability to recognize new antigens introduced to the body. Thymocyte numbers decrease with aging, which results in a decline in immune function and the ability to fight new diseases [5]. Mouse and human thymocytes express GHS-R1a, and ablation of GHS-R1a in mice results in accelerated age-dependent thymocyte death [5]. Interestingly, ghrelin treatment was able to prevent such accelerated thymocyte loss with age [5], and inflammation by cytokines [59]. Thus, GHS-R1a agonism could potentially extend the longevity of the immune system and overall capacity to overcome disease and inflammation.

Hip fracture is another age-related disorder that has been linked to the gradual loss of muscle and bones due to low GH signaling. Hip fracture usually results in further mobility loss and a rapid decrease in health due to complications. Since MK0677 accelerated hip fracture recovery in 60-year-old patients [60] and also has GH-stimulating properties, GHS-R1a agonism could help in both hip fracture treatment and prevention.

Other Ghrelin Receptors

Interestingly, des-acyl ghrelin has been shown to oppose the physiological effects of ghrelin. Baldanzi et al. [61] performed a series of binding assays that revealed a novel receptor with the same affinity for des-acyl ghrelin as for acyl-ghrelin in a heart cell line that, according to their studies, do not express the GHS-R1a. Observations like these, as well as those in vivo, such as ghrelin deletion improving glucose metabolism in mice [2], have suggested there is a second receptor for ghrelin. These findings have triggered an ongoing quest to identify potentially both a des-acyl ghrelin receptor and/or a second ghrelin receptor. Some studies show evidence of ghrelin binding in muscle and bone cells [62], and ghrelin actions in chondrocytes indicate that ghrelin activates a receptor that couples to $G_{\alpha s}$ and a cAMP regulated pathway [63]. However, a second receptor has not yet been cloned and, thus, the existence of such a receptor remains an open question in the field.

Conclusion

In summary, GPCRs are the largest group of receptors present at the plasma membrane. They are the ‘gate’ to cell signaling modulation and thus have been exploited pharmacologically to treat many diseases. However, one receptor can be expressed in many tissues and different areas of the brain, making it difficult to isolate the effects of a global agonist or antagonist. The ability of the GHS-R1a to dimerize with other receptors will likely allow for new treatments that selectively activate only specific dimers, and thus, only in certain subsets of neurons. This will modulate signaling in a much more targeted fashion, resulting in a smaller number of negative side effects. As we have reviewed, MK0677 and anamorelin are two drugs that could potentially treat ailments, including cachexia, neurodegeneration, inflammation and cardiac function. GHS-R1a antagonists have not been used in humans to date, but as we have described in this chapter, such antagonists may be beneficial for other neurological conditions, as well as for improving insulin sensitivity and glucose homeostasis in type 2 diabetes.

References

1 Diano S, et al: Ghrelin controls hippocampal spine synapse density and memory performance. Nat Neurosci 2006;9:381–388.
2 Sun Y, Asnicar M, Smith RG: Central and peripheral roles of ghrelin on glucose homeostasis. Neuroendocrinology 2007;86:215–228.
3 Andrews ZB, et al: Ghrelin promotes and protects nigrostriatal dopamine function via a UCP2-dependent mitochondrial mechanism. J Neurosci 2009;29: 14057–14065.
4 Albarran-Zeckler RG, Sun Y, Smith RG: Physiological roles revealed by ghrelin and ghrelin receptor deficient mice. Peptides 2011;32:2229–2235.
5 Dixit VD, et al: Ghrelin promotes thymopoiesis during aging. J Clin Invest 2007;117:2778–2790.
6 Abizaid A, et al: Ghrelin modulates the activity and synaptic input organization of midbrain dopamine neurons while promoting appetite. J Clin Invest 2006;116:3229–3239.
7 Albarran-Zeckler RG, Brantley AF, Smith RG: Growth hormone secretagogue receptor (GHS-R1a) knockout mice exhibit improved spatial memory and deficits in contextual memory. Behav Brain Res 2012;232:13–19.
8 Garcia JM, Friend J, Allen S: Therapeutic potential of anamorelin, a novel, oral ghrelin mimetic, in patients with cancer-related cachexia: a multicenter, randomized, double-blind, crossover, pilot study. Support Care Cancer 2013;21:129–137.
9 Egecioglu E, et al: Ghrelin increases intake of rewarding food in rodents. Addict Biol 2010;15:304–311.
10 Jiang H, Betancourt L, Smith RG: Ghrelin amplifies dopamine signaling by cross talk involving formation of growth hormone secretagogue receptor/dopamine receptor subtype 1 heterodimers. Mol Endocrinol 2006;20:1772–1785.
11 Kern A, et al: Apo-ghrelin receptor forms heteromers with DRD2 in hypothalamic neurons and is essential for anorexigenic effects of DRD2 agonism. Neuron 2012;73:317–332.
12 Milligan G: G protein-coupled receptor heterodimers: pharmacology, function and relevance to drug discovery. Drug Discovery Today 2006;11:541–549.
13 Smith RG, et al: Modulation of pulsatile GH release through a novel receptor in hypothalamus and pituitary gland. Rec Prog Horm Res 1996;51:261–286.
14 Smith RG, et al: A nonpeptidyl growth hormone secretagogue. Science 1993;260:1640–1643.
15 Bowers CY, et al: On the in vitro and in vivo activity of a new synthetic hexapeptide that acts on the pituitary to specifically release growth hormone. Endocrinology 1984;114:1537–1545.
16 Smith RG, et al: Mechanism of action of GHRP-6 and nonpeptidyl growth hormone secretagogues; in Bercu BB, Walker RF (eds): Growth Hormone Secretagogues, Serono Symposia. New York, Springer, 1996, pp 147–163.
17 Howard AD, et al: A receptor in pituitary and hypothalamus that functions in growth hormone release. Science 1996;273:974–977.
18 Honda K, et al: An electrophysiological and morphological investigation of the projections of growth hormone-releasing peptide-6-responsive neurons in the rat arcuate nucleus to the median eminence and to the paraventricular nucleus. Neuroscience 1999; 90:875–883.
19 Liu B, Garcia EA, Korbonits M: Genetic studies on the ghrelin, growth hormone secretagogue receptor (GHSR) and ghrelin *O*-acyl transferase (GOAT) genes. Peptides 2011;32:2191–2207.
20 Kojima M, et al: Ghrelin is a growth-hormone-releasing acylated peptide from stomach. Nature 1999; 402:656–660.
21 Yang J, et al: Identification of the acyltransferase that octanoylates ghrelin, an appetite-stimulating peptide hormone. Cell 2008;132:387–396.
22 Gutierrez JA, et al: Ghrelin octanoylation mediated by an orphan lipid transferase. Proc Natl Acad Sci USA 2008;105:6320–6325.

23 Kirchner H, et al: Ghrelin and PYY in the regulation of energy balance and metabolism: lessons from mouse mutants. Am J Physiology Endocrinol Metab 2010;298:E909–E919.
24 Nakazato M, et al: A role for ghrelin in the central regulation of feeding. Nature 2001;409:194–198.
25 Smith RG, et al: A new orphan receptor involved in pulsatile growth hormone release. Trends Endocrinol Metab 1999;10:128–135.
26 Leung PK, et al: The truncated ghrelin receptor polypeptide (GHS-R1b) acts as a dominant-negative mutant of the ghrelin receptor. Cell Signal 2007;19: 1011–1022.
27 Chow KB, et al: The truncated ghrelin receptor polypeptide (GHS-R1b) is localized in the endoplasmic reticulum where it forms heterodimers with ghrelin receptors (GHS-R1a) to attenuate their cell surface expression. Mol Cell Endocrinol 2012;348:247–254.
28 Nagaya N, et al: Hemodynamic and hormonal effects of human ghrelin in healthy volunteers. Am J Physiol Regul Integr Comp Physiol 2001;280:R1483–R1487.
29 Sun Y, et al: Characterization of adult ghrelin and ghrelin receptor knockout mice under positive and negative energy balance. Endocrinology 2008;149: 843–850.
30 Tesauro M, et al: Metabolic and cardiovascular effects of ghrelin. Int J Pept 2010;2010 pii:864342.
31 Svensson J, et al: Two-Month treatment of obese subjects with the oral growth hormone (GH) secretagogue MK-677 increases GH secretion, fat-free mass, and energy expenditure. J Clin Endocrinol Metab 1998;83:362–369.
32 Chapman IM, et al: Stimulation of the growth hormone (GH)-insulin-like growth factor-I axis by daily oral administration of a GH secretagogue (MK-0677) in healthy elderly subjects. J Clin Endocrinol Metab 1996;81:4249–4257.
33 Sun Y, et al: Ghrelin stimulation of growth hormone release and appetite is mediated through the growth hormone secretagogue receptor. Proc Natl Acad Sci USA 2004;101:4679–4684.
34 Zigman JM, et al: Mice lacking ghrelin receptors resist the development of diet-induced obesity. J Clin Invest 2005;115:3564–3572.
35 Sun Y, et al: Ablation of ghrelin improves the diabetic but not obese phenotype of ob/ob mice. Cell Metab 2006;3:379–386.
36 Muzzin P, et al: Correction of obesity and diabetes in genetically obese mice by leptin gene therapy. Proc Natl Acad Sci USA 1996;93:14804–14808.
37 Cowley MA, et al: The distribution and mechanism of action of ghrelin in the CNS demonstrates a novel hypothalamic circuit regulating energy homeostasis. Neuron 2003;37:649–661.
38 Ellis J, et al: Orexin-1 receptor-cannabinoid CB1 receptor heterodimerization results in both ligand-dependent and -independent coordinated alterations of receptor localization and function. J Biol Chem 2006;281:38812–38824.
39 Rediger A, et al: Mutually opposite signal modulation by hypothalamic heterodimerization of ghrelin and melanocortin-3 receptors. J Biol Chem 2011; 286:39623–39631.
40 Ortiz O, et al: Associative learning and CA3-CA1 synaptic plasticity are impaired in D1R null, Drd1a–/– mice and in hippocampal siRNA silenced Drd1a mice. J Neurosci 2010;30:12288–12300.
41 Wellman PJ, Hollas CN, Elliott AE: Systemic ghrelin sensitizes cocaine-induced hyperlocomotion in rats. Regul Pept 2008;146:33–37.
42 Jerlhag E, et al: The alcohol-induced locomotor stimulation and accumbal dopamine release is suppressed in ghrelin knockout mice. Alcohol 2011;45: 341–347.
43 Jerlhag E, et al: Ghrelin receptor antagonism attenuates cocaine- and amphetamine-induced locomotor stimulation, accumbal dopamine release, and conditioned place preference. Psychopharmacology (Berl) 2010;211:415–422.
44 Wei YH, et al: Oxidative damage and mutation to mitochondrial DNA and age-dependent decline of mitochondrial respiratory function. Ann NY Acad Sci 1998;854:155–170.
45 Massaad CA: Neuronal and vascular oxidative stress in Alzheimer's disease. Curr Neuropharmacol 2011; 9:662–673.
46 Moon M, et al: Neuroprotective effect of ghrelin in the 1-methyl-4-phenyl-1,2,3,6-tetrahydropyridine mouse model of Parkinson's disease by blocking microglial activation. Neurotox Res 2009;15:332–347.
47 Jiang H, et al: Ghrelin antagonizes MPTP-induced neurotoxicity to the dopaminergic neurons in mouse substantia nigra. Exp Neurol 2008;212:532–537.
48 Richard D, et al: Uncoupling protein 2 in the brain: distribution and function. Biochem Soc Trans 2001; 29:812–817.
49 Chung H, et al: Ghrelin suppresses tunicamycin- or thapsigargin-triggered endoplasmic reticulum stress-mediated apoptosis in primary cultured rat cortical neuronal cells. Endocr J 2011;58:409–420.
50 Chow KB, Cheng CH, Wise H: Anti-inflammatory activity of ghrelin in human carotid artery cells. Inflammation 2009;32:402–409.
51 Enomoto M, et al: Cardiovascular and hormonal effects of subcutaneous administration of ghrelin, a novel growth hormone-releasing peptide, in healthy humans. Clin Sci (Lond) 2003;105:431–435.
52 Nagaya N, et al: Chronic administration of ghrelin improves left ventricular dysfunction and attenuates development of cardiac cachexia in rats with heart failure. Circulation 2001;104:1430–1435.

53 Palus S, et al: Ghrelin and its analogues, BIM-28131 and BIM-28125, improve body weight and regulate the expression of MuRF-1 and MAFbx in a rat heart failure model. PLoS One 2011;6:e26865.
54 Klocke R, et al: Surgical animal models of heart failure related to coronary heart disease. Cardiovasc Res 2007;74:29–38.
55 Nagaya N, et al: Effects of ghrelin administration on left ventricular function, exercise capacity, and muscle wasting in patients with chronic heart failure. Circulation 2004;110:3674–3679.
56 Garcia JM, et al: Active ghrelin levels and active to total ghrelin ratio in cancer-induced cachexia. J Clin Endocrinol Metab 2005;90:2920–2926.
57 Nagaya N, et al: Elevated circulating level of ghrelin in cachexia associated with chronic heart failure: relationships between ghrelin and anabolic/catabolic factors. Circulation 2001;104:2034–2038.
58 Garcia JM, et al: Ghrelin prevents cisplatin-induced mechanical hyperalgesia and cachexia. Endocrinology 2008;149:455–460.
59 Dixit VD, et al: Ghrelin inhibits leptin- and activation-induced proinflammatory cytokine expression by human monocytes and T cells. J Clin Invest 2004;114:57–66.
60 Adunsky A, et al: MK-0677 (ibutamoren mesylate) for the treatment of patients recovering from hip fracture: a multicenter, randomized, placebo-controlled phase IIb study. Arch Gerontol Geriatr 2011;53:183–189.
61 Baldanzi G, et al: Ghrelin and des-acyl ghrelin inhibit cell death in cardiomyocytes and endothelial cells through ERK1/2 and PI 3-kinase/AKT. J Cell Biol 2002;159:1029–1037.
62 Filigheddu N, et al: Ghrelin and des-acyl ghrelin promote differentiation and fusion of C2C12 skeletal muscle cells. Mol Biol Cell 2007;18:986–994.
63 Caminos JE, et al: The endogenous growth hormone secretagogue (ghrelin) is synthesized and secreted by chondrocytes. Endocrinology 2005;146:1285–1292.

Roy G. Smith, PhD
Department of Metabolism and Aging, The Scripps Research Institute, Scripps Florida
130 Scripps Way #3B3
Jupiter, FL 33458 (USA)
E-Mail rgsmith@scripps.edu

Benso A, Casanueva FF, Ghigo E, Granata A (eds): The Ghrelin System.
Endocr Dev. Basel, Karger, 2013, vol 25, pp 16–24 (DOI: 10.1159/000346039)

Discovery of Ghrelin *O*-Acyltransferase

Haneesha Mohan · Suraj Unniappan

Department of Veterinary Biomedical Sciences, Laboratory of Integrative Neuroendocrinology, Western College of Veterinary Medicine, University of Saskatchewan, Saskatoon, SAS, Canada

Abstract

Ghrelin is a gut hormone with potent orexigenic and growth hormone release stimulatory effects, and is the first known endogenous ligand of the growth hormone secretagogue receptor. A notable feature of ghrelin is that it carries an acyl group, in most cases an octanoyl group, in the third serine. While it has been shown that the acylation is critical for the majority of ghrelin functions, the mechanisms of acylation of ghrelin remained poorly understood. In 2008, it was discovered that ghrelin *O*-acyltransferase (GOAT) is the enzyme responsible for acylating ghrelin. GOAT is highly conserved from zebrafish to humans. It is most abundant in the stomach and pancreas. GOAT mRNA expression is regulated by energy balance, being upregulated by energy restriction and downregulated by energy abundance. GOAT attenuation using synthetic inhibitors enhances insulin secretion and reduces body weight. GOAT inhibitors are currently being developed for the treatment of metabolic disorders. In addition to its ghrelin mediated effects, GOAT is also known to directly regulate bile acid secretion. The discovery of GOAT helped to redefine the ghrelin research field and enabled the development of another target molecule for potential therapies aimed to prevent/treat diabetes and obesity.

From the U-Factor to GOAT

In the 1970s, Cyril Bowers proposed that an unknown endogenous factor (U-factor), in addition to the growth hormone-releasing hormone (GHRH) and somatostatin, regulates growth hormone (GH) release from the pituitary [1, 2]. The Bowers lab synthesized the first growth hormone secretagogue (GHS), growth hormone-releasing peptide-6 that has potent GH-releasing effects [2]. Following this invention, many researchers including Bowers, and scientists from the Merck Research Laboratories pioneered and developed a variety of synthetic GHSs of peptidyl and nonpeptidyl origin [3]. The GHS field rapidly expanded in the next 20 years, and a main focus was to identify the receptor(s) to which the GHSs bind. In 1996, almost 20 years following the proposition of the U-factor, an orphan receptor to which GHSs bind was discovered by Howard et al. [4] from the Merck Research Laboratories. This receptor which is most abundant in the pituitary and hypothalamus was named the growth hormone secretagogue receptor (GHS-R) and is currently called as the ghrelin receptor. The identification of the receptor led to the search for an endogenous ligand, and in 1999, Masayasu Kojima and colleagues from Kenji Kangawa's laboratory discovered an endogenous ligand for the GHS-R [5]. This peptide was named ghrelin, reflecting its ability to promote GH secretion and growth. After cholecystokinin that has a sulfonylation [6], ghrelin is the second hormone known to have a unique modification named acylation [5]. It is also the only known gut-derived orexigen [5]. The addition of an acyl group (predominantly octanoyl group) is essential for the majority of ghrelin biological actions [7]. However, the details of acylation, especially the enzyme that facilitates this modification remained elusive. In 2008, a decade after the discovery of ghrelin, two concurrent papers reported the discovery of ghrelin *O*-acyltransferase (GOAT) [8, 9]. This discovery is the most recent major advance in the ghrelin research field. The ground breaking discoveries of Bowers and a number of other researchers, Kangawa and colleagues, and the Goldstein and Gutierrez groups constitute the major events in the journey from GHS to acylated ghrelin. A historical timeline of events in the GHS/ghrelin research is shown in figure 1a. The focus of this chapter is to succinctly discuss the discovery of GOAT and the notable progress in GOAT research to date.

Discovery of GOAT

In the original research that reported the discovery of ghrelin, Kojima and colleagues used mass spectroscopy analysis to provide the initial evidence for the acylation of ghrelin [5]. They found that the third residue serine in ghrelin is modified by an octanoyl group. Addition of this acyl group (acylation/esterification) is critical for the growth hormone releasing activity and several other actions of ghrelin [5]. However, the process of acylation, as well as the possible enzyme(s) behind this process remained unsolved. Meanwhile, in the unrelated area of enzyme research, several new ideas were shaping up. Specifically, Hofmann [10] using novel combinations of bioinformatics tools identified a family of *O*-acyltransferases that catalyses the *O*-acylation reaction. These findings were rooted in genetic studies performed earlier on *Drosophilia*, based on a gene called *porcupine* [11]. *Porcupine* has conserved regions that is also found in many membrane bound hydrophobic enzymes that are involved in translocating long chain fatty acids to membrane bound hydroxyl receptors. These enzymes were called membrane-bound *O*-acyltransferases (MBOATs) [11]. This advance in the MBOAT research eventually led to the discovery of what we know now as the ghrelin *O*-acyltransferase (GOAT).

GOAT was identified independently by two research groups, and was reported to the scientific community in two elegant articles [8, 9] published months apart in

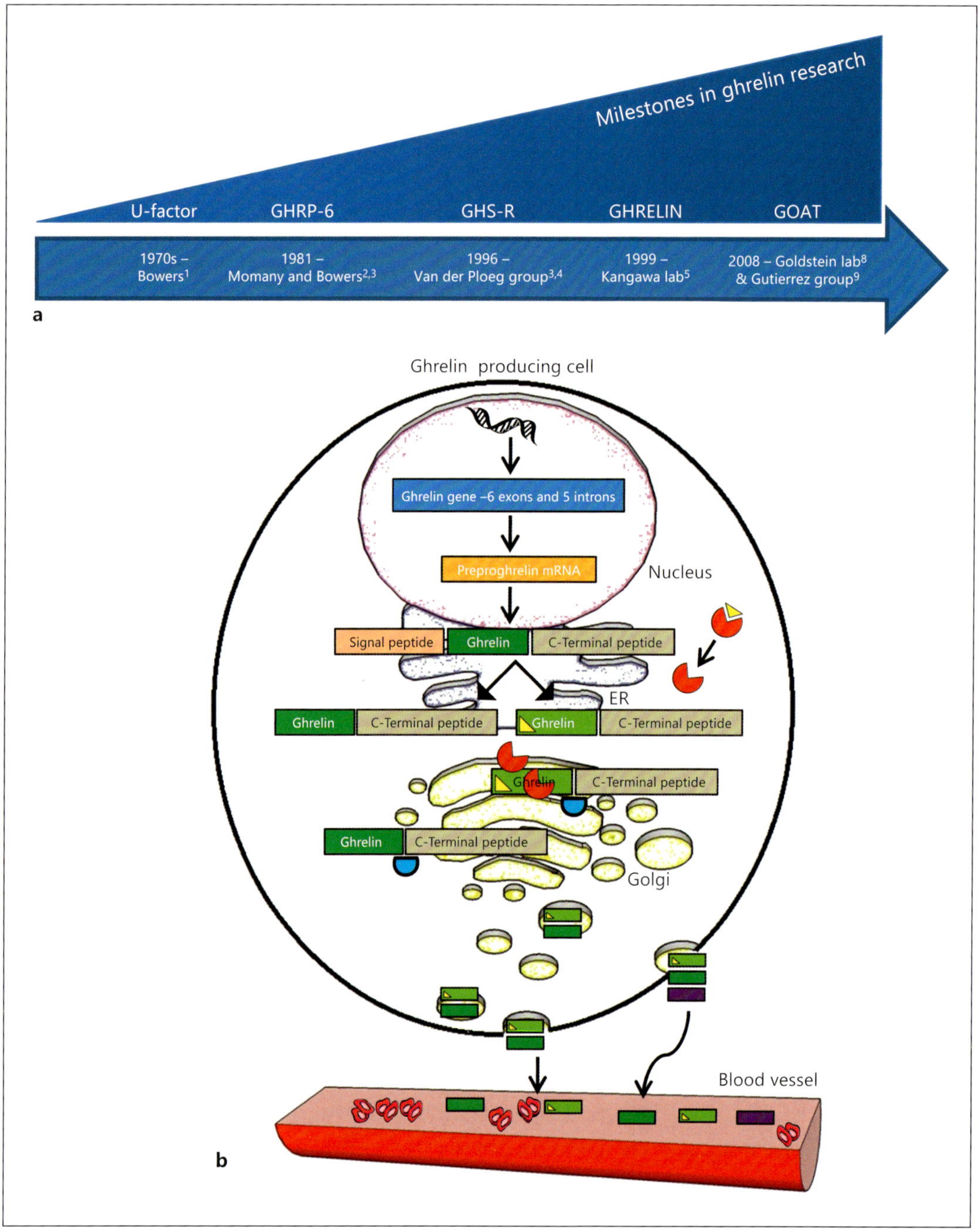

Fig. 1. a Summary of milestones in GHS, ghrelin, GHS-R and GOAT research. The triangle shows the sequence of events that expanded the GHS/ghrelin research field. The year of the major findings and the corresponding author of the major article reporting the findings is named underneath the triangle, inside the arrow. The references are provided in superscript and the full citations are available in the reference list. **b** Schematic Illustration of the posttranslational processing of the ghrelin gene. Preproghrelin mRNA is transcribed from the ghrelin gene in the nucleus. A precursor peptide is

2008. In the article that came first in the public domain, Yang et al. [8] determined that the mouse genome encodes for 16 membrane-bound MBOAT protein sequences produced by 11 genes. Later studies on cultured endocrine cells lines co-transfected with preproghrelin sequence and MBOATs revealed that one of these MBOATs catalyzed the octanoylation of ghrelin. This MBOAT facilitating ghrelin acylation was then named GOAT [8]. There were 11 catalytic regions that are highly conserved in all 16 MBOAT sequences in the mouse genome. The conserved regions contain the putative asparagine and histidine residues that are thought to take part in the catalytic reactions [8]. A series of transfection experiments demonstrated that GOAT-dependent octanylation of ghrelin in three different murine endocrine cell lines. When mouse pituitary AtT-20 cells, rat insulinoma INS-1 cells, and mouse insulinoma MIN-6 cells were cotransfected with preproghrelin and GOAT, acylated ghrelin was produced. Mutation of the serine at position 3 to alanine prevented the acyl modification of ghrelin by GOAT, indicating that the presence of third serine is essential for GOAT-dependent octanylation of ghrelin [8]. Additional studies demonstrated that proghrelin is octanoylated before it reaches the Golgi where prohormone convertases 1/3 (PC 1/3) posttranslationally cleave pro-ghrelin to form mature ghrelin [12]. This suggests that GOAT is present in the endoplasmic reticulum promoting acylation on proghrelin before being translocated to the Golgi [8]. Figure 1b provides an overview of cellular events leading to the synthesis and secretion of ghrelin. Overall, these results by Yang et al. [8] provide the first reported experimental evidence for GOAT.

Meanwhile, the second group led by Gutierrez et al. [9] studied ghrelin octanoylation in vitro using human medullary thyroid carcinoma (TT) cells to identify which member of the MBOAT family is involved in ghrelin acylation. Less than 10% of ghrelin secreted by the TT cells were acylated, leading them to think that there is a low expression of the acylating machinery in TT cells [9]. Silencing the GOAT gene in the TT cells using several GOAT specific siRNAs resulted in an inhibition of ghrelin acylation. Gene silencing of other MBOAT members present in the TT cells did not affect ghrelin octanoylation, implicating solely GOAT in the acylation of ghrelin. In addition, HEK-293 cells that neither express ghrelin nor GOAT, when cotransfected with preproghrelin and GOAT, started secreting octanoylated ghrelin [9]. Further experiments conclusively showed that ghrelin octanoylation was only achieved with GOAT, although these cells were coexpressed with other members of the MBOAT

formed in the ER following the translation of preproghrelin mRNA which consists of a signal peptide, mature ghrelin and a C-terminal peptide. After the cleavage of the signal sequence by signal peptide peptidase, pro-ghrelin is produced either as acylated proghrelin or unacylated proghrelin. Acylated proghrelin is produced when GOAT ( ) in the ER translocates octanoyl-CoA ( ) to acylate pro-ghrelin before it reaches the Golgi where prohormone convertases 1/3 (PC 1/3;) posttranslationally cleave acylated or unacylated pro-ghrelin to form mature ghrelin forms. Acylated ( ), unacylated ( ), and other shorter forms of ghrelin ( ) are packaged into vesicles from the Golgi and released into the blood circulation.

family, including MBOAT1, MBOAT2, MBOAT3, MBOAT5, human-BB1, porcupine, and FKSG89. The replacement of the conserved histidine residue in GOAT to alanine (H338A) inhibited its activity, demonstrating further that GOAT is a member of the MBOAT protein family [9]. Also, HEK-293 cell medium treated with a variety of substrate lipids, including tetradecanoic acid caused acylation of ghrelin. This suggests that GOAT could use a selection of fatty acids in addition to octanoic and decanoic acid to acylate ghrelin [9].

Since there is very high similarity in GOAT proteins across many vertebrate, Gutierrez et al. [9], conducted additional studies to determine whether the function of GOAT is conserved across species. HEK-293 cells were transfected with rat, mouse or zebrafish GOAT resulted in successful octanoylation of human ghrelin, demonstrating that the function of GOAT is highly conserved across vertebrates [9]. Further studies on GOAT gene knockout mice, confirmed that GOAT is the critical lipid acyl transferase for acylating ghrelin as there was no detectable levels of octanoylated ghrelin in the GOAT knockout mice compared to wild-type controls [9]. Collectively, these results from Gutierrez and colleagues [9] confirmed Yang et al.'s [8] findings and strengthened the notion that GOAT is the enzyme responsible for ghrelin acylation. More recent studies by Ohgusu et al. [13] discovered that peptides as short as four amino acids consisting of an unblocked N-terminal region are acyl-modified by GOAT. Their studies demonstrated that GOAT prefers n-hexanoyl-CoA as the acyl donor instead of n-octanoyl CoA [13]. Thus far, ghrelin modified by various forms of lipids were reported [7].

Pattern of GOAT mRNA and Protein Expression in Tissues

Yang et al. found that the highest levels of GOAT mRNA expression were limited to the stomach and intestine followed by the testis of mice [8]. In rats, GOAT mRNA expression is also identified in the hypothalamus, stomach, intestine, ovary, serum, placenta, muscle, heart, and adrenal glands [14]. Gutierrez et al. [9] demonstrated that in humans GOAT transcript levels is most abundant in the stomach and pancreas. From these results, it is highly evident that the stomach is the main tissue for acyl ghrelin production and changes in the secretion of acylated ghrelin can modulate changes in metabolism of many species. GOAT-immunopositive ghrelin cells found in mice (95%) stomach are higher in comparison to rats (56%) [15]. GOAT mRNA and protein are present in the whole pancreas, isolated islets and INS-1 cells. GOAT immunopositive cells are mainly localized in the periphery of rat islets [16]. In diet-induced obese (DIO) and ob/ob mice, it was found that the GOAT mRNA levels were decreased in the pituitary in comparison to the hypothalamus. Although GOAT mRNA expression increased in the pituitary after a 24 h fast, and it increased in the hypothalamus at 48 h of fasting. GOAT is also expressed in the hypothalamus and pituitary of mice [17]. Overall, GOAT appears to be predominantly expressed in the gut, brain and the pancreas, three tissues that play major roles in feeding and energy homeostasis.

GOAT expression is modulated by nutrition. For instance, mice in a state of negative energy balance, or fasted for 24 or 48 h have shown increased GOAT expression, while, in a positive energy balance state, GOAT expression decreases [17, 18]. However, in another study performed by Gonzalez et al. [14] there was no change in GOAT mRNA expression after 48 h of fasting in rats. Meanwhile, they found that chronic malnutrition achieved by 70% restriction in food intake for 21 days led to an increase in GOAT expression in the gastric mucosa [14]. This is contradictory to another study where 35% of dietary food restriction for 5 months significantly reduced the levels of GOAT expression in the stomach [19]. Furthermore, a study by Kirchner et al. [20] found that when mice are fed ad libitum, expression of GOAT was evidently high but decreased after 12, 24, 36, and 48 h of fasting. While variations exist between tissues, species and strains, it is important to learn that metabolic status influences the expression of GOAT. These data suggest that GOAT is possibly linked to metabolic regulation.

Implications of GOAT in Metabolism and Metabolic Disorders

As GOAT is co-expressed with ghrelin in the pancreas, GOAT has been implicated in the regulation of insulin secretion and glucose metabolism. GOAT knockout mice fasted for 16 hours have increased insulin secretion and improved glucose tolerance [21]. In addition, GOAT knock-out mice provided with a 60% caloric restriction diet have shown to develop severe hypoglycemia, with 2% reduction in body fat compared to wild type mice and were morbid after 7 days [21]. When these mice were infused with ghrelin or GH, their blood glucose reached normal levels and prevented death. These studies suggest that caloric deficiency can modulate the expression of ghrelin and GH levels in the absence of GOAT and thus implicate its role in glucose metabolism [21]. Recently, GOAT has been associated with anorexia nervosa as a result of genetic variations found in the GOAT gene [22].

Ghrelin has been actively pursued as a potential antiobesity target. Discovery of GOAT led to a new line to translational research aimed to develop GOAT inhibitors. The idea behind this approach is to inhibit GOAT, thereby inhibiting synthesis of active ghrelin, which is involved in stimulating a positive energy balance and inhibiting insulin secretion. Thus far, two effective GOAT inhibitors have been validated. The first one developed by Yang et al. [23] is a potent inhibitor of GOAT activity in vitro. The first and rather extensive in vivo characterization of a different type of GOAT inhibitor named GO-CoA-Tat was reported by Barnett et al. [24]. In vivo administration of GO-CoA-Tat resulted in a significant reduction in body weight, an increase in glucose-stimulated insulin secretion (GSIS). This effect on insulin secretion is mediated by inhibiting UCP2, which has negative effects on GSIS. It was also found that islet

GOAT mRNA expression is inhibited by insulin, and that the insulin effects on GOAT are mediated via the PI3 kinase/AkT pathway and by inhibiting the GOAT promoter activity [25]. These results clearly indicate an important role for GOAT on insulin synthesis and secretion from pancreatic islets. Collectively, the data obtained from GOAT null mice and studies using GOAT inhibitors clearly indicate a role for GOAT in the regulation of energy balance. These metabolic effects of GOAT appear to be mediated mainly via its modulatory roles on ghrelin. At least one study suggests that the intraislet ghrelin/GOAT is not responsible for modulating insulin secretion. Bando et al. [26] developed a new mouse strain that has intraislet overexpression of both ghrelin and GOAT under the rat insulin promoter. These mice have normal portal vein ghrelin levels, glucose homeostasis, insulin levels and islet morphology. A suggested possibility is that the islet beta cells are unable to make acylated ghrelin due to the absence of critical cellular components that are present in the gastric ghrelin cells. Further studies are required to determine the tissue specific presence and function of the GOAT.

GOAT is the only known enzyme that acylates ghrelin. However, it is possible that GOAT might have other effects on homeostasis, especially by acting on other hormones or physiological processes. In line with this possibility, a very recent study by Kang et al. [27] showed that GOAT has a crucial role in the regulation of bile acid reabsorption. GOAT null mice exhibited an approximately 2.5-fold increase in secondary bile acids. GOAT null mice have an increase in the expression of illeal sodium-dependent bile acid transporter mRNA and protein in both the biliary tract and the gastrointestinal (GI) tract. A similar ~10-fold increase in the solute carrier family 5 (Slc5a12), a sodium/glucose cotransporter was also detected in the small intestine and bile duct. This study provides the first glimpse of GOAT effects unrelated to ghrelin. More studies are essential to identify the physiology of GOAT and complete functional implications of GOAT absence.

Conclusions

The discovery of GOAT further strengthened and expanded the ghrelin research field. First, it provided certainty to the mechanisms underlying the unique acyl modification found in ghrelin. Second, it opened the door for an important research area on GOAT, a molecule that has to be considered while studying ghrelin biology. Third, GOAT provides an opportunity to modulate the ghrelinergic system for potential therapeutic outcomes. Specifically, GOAT is now a target molecule for developing possible therapies for obesity and diabetes as it is critical for the metabolic and insulinostatic properties of ghrelin. Collectively, the identification of GOAT redefined the ghrelinergic system and its functional significance. Future research on the ghrelinergic system, including GOAT is expected to provide more clarity to the findings on this interesting research field. It is also important to pursue research aimed to elucidate specific functions of GOAT that are independent of ghrelin.

Acknowledgments

The research in the author's laboratory is supported by the Natural Sciences and Engineering Research Council of Canada, Saskatchewan Health Research Foundation (SHRF) and the Canadian Institute of Health Research (CIHR). Suraj Unniappan is a CIHR New Investigator, and a recipient of the Early Research award from the Ministry of Research and Innovation of Ontario.

References

1 Deghenghi R: Structural requirements of growth hormone secretagogues; in Bercu BB, Walker RF (eds): Growth Hormone Secretagogues in Clinical Practice. New York, Marcel Dekker, 1998, pp 27–35.

2 Bowers CY, Reynolds GA, Momany FA: New advances on the regulation of growth hormone (GH) secretion. Int J Neurol 1984;18:188–205.

3 Smith RG, Sun Y, Betancourt L, Asnicar M: Growth hormone secretagogues: prospects and potential pitfalls. Best Pract Res Clin Endocrinol Metab 2004;18: 333–347

4 Howard AD, Feighner SD, Cully DF, Arena JP, Liberator PA, Rosenblum CI, Hamelin M, Hreniuk DL, Palyha OC, Anderson J, Paress PS, Diaz C, Chou M, Liu KK, McKee KK, Pong SS, Chaung LY, Elbrecht A, Dashkevicz M, Heavens R, Rigby M, Sirinathsinghji DJ, Dean DC, Melillo DG, Patchett AA, Nargund R, Griffin PR, DeMartino JA, Gupta SK, Schaeffer JM, Smith RG, Van der Ploeg LH: A receptor in pituitary and hypothalamus that functions in growth hormone release. Science. 1996;273:974–977

5 Kojima M, Hosoda H, Date Y, Nakazato M, Matsuo H, Kangawa K: Ghrelin is a growth-hormone-releasing acylated peptide from stomach. Nature 1999;402: 656–660.

6 Smith GP: The therapeutic potential of cholecystokinin. Int J Obes 1984;8:35–38.

7 Kojima M, Kangawa K: Ghrelin: Structure and function. Physiol Rev 2005;85:495–522.

8 Yang J, Brown MS, Liang G, Grishin NV, Goldstein JL: Identification of the acyltransferase that octanoylates ghrelin, an appetite-stimulating peptide hormone. Cell 2008;132:387–396.

9 Gutierrez JA, Solenberg PJ, Perkins DR, Willency JA, Knierman MD, Jin Z, Witcher DR, Luo S, Onyia JE, Hale JE: Ghrelin octanoylation mediated by an orphan lipid transferase. Proc Natl Acad Sci USA 2008; 105:6320–6325.

10 Hofmann, K: A superfamily of membrane-bound O-acyltransferases with implications for Wnt signaling. Trends Biochem Sci 2000;25:111–112.

11 Kadowaki T, Wilder E, Klingensmith J, Zachary K, Perrimon N: The segment polarity gene porcupine encodes a putative multitrans-membrane protein involved in Wingless processing. Genes Dev 1996;10: 3116–3128.

12 Zhu X, Cao Y, Voogd K, Steiner DF: On the processing of proghrelin to ghrelin. J Biol Chem 2006;281: 38867–38870.

13 Ohgusu H, Shirouzu K, Nakamura Y, Nakashima Y, Ida T, Sato T, Kojima M: Ghrelin *O*-acyltransferase (GOAT) has a preference for n-hexanoyl-CoA over n-octanoyl-CoA as an acyl donor. Biochem Biophys Res Commun 2009;386:153–158.

14 González CR, Vázquez MJ, López M, Diéguez C: Influence of chronic undernutrition and leptin on GOAT mRNA levels in rat stomach mucosa. J Mol Endocrinol 2008;41:415–421.

15 Stengel A, Goebel M, Wang L, Taché Y, Sachs G, Lambrecht NW: Differential distribution of ghrelin-*O*-acyltransferase (GOAT) immunoreactive cells in the mouse International Journal of Peptides 5 and rat gastric oxyntic mucosa. Biochem Biophys Res Commun 2010;392:67–71.

16 An W, Li Y, Xu G, Zhao J, Xiang X, Ding L, Li J, Guan Y, Wang X, Tang C, Li X, Mulholland M, Zhang W: Modulation of ghrelin *O*-acyltransferase expression in pancreatic islets. Cell Physiol Biochem 2010;26: 707–716.

17 Gahete MD, Córdoba-Chacón J, Salvatori R, Castaño JP, Kineman RD, Luque RM: Metabolic regulation of ghrelin *O*-acyl transferase (GOAT) expression in the mouse hypothalamus, pituitary, and stomach. Mol Cell Endocrinol 2010;317:154–160.

18 Xu G, Li Y, An W, Li S, Guan Y, Wang N, Tang C, Wang X, Zhu Y, Li X, Mulholland MW, Zhang W: Gastric mammalian target of rapamycin signaling regulates ghrelin production and food intake. Endocrinology 2009;150:3637–3644.

19 Reimer RA, Maurer AD, Lau DC, Auer RN: Long-term dietary restriction influences plasma ghrelin and GOAT mRNA level in rats. Physiol Behav 2010; 99:605–610.

20 Kirchner H, Gutierrez JA, Solenberg PJ, Pfluger PT, Czyzyk TA, Willency JA, Schürmann A, Joost HG, Jandacek RJ, Hale JE, Heiman ML, Tschöp MH: GOAT links dietary lipids with the endocrine control of energy balance. Nat Med 2009;15:741–745.
21 Zhao TJ, Liang G, Li RL, Xie X, Sleeman MW, Murphy AJ, Valenzuela DM, Yancopoulos GD, Goldstein JL, Brown MS: Ghrelin *O*-acyltransferase (GOAT) is essential for growth hormone-mediated survival of calorie-restricted mice. Proc Natl Acad Sci USA 2010;107:7467–7472.
22 Soriano-Guillén L, Barrios V, Campos-Barros A, Argente J: Ghrelin levels in obesity and anorexia nervosa: effect of weight reduction or recuperation. J Pediatr 2004;144:36–42.
23 Yang Y, Zhao TJ, Goldstein JL, Brown MS: Inhibition of ghrelin *O*-acyltransferase (GOAT) by octanoylated pentapeptides. Proc Natl Acad Sci USA 2008;105:10750–10755.
24 Barnett BP, Hwang Y, Taylor MS, Kirchner H, Pfluger PT, Bernard V, Lin YY, Bowers EM, Mukherjee C, Song WJ, Longo PA, Leahy DJ, Hussain MA, Tschöp MH, Boeke JD, Cole PA: Glucose and weight control in mice with a designed ghrelin *O*-acyltransferase inhibitor. Science 2010;330:1689–1692.
25 An W, Li Y, Xu G, Zhao J, Xiang X, Ding L, Li J, Guan Y, Wang X, Tang C, Li X, Mulholland M, Zhang W: Modulation of ghrelin *O*-acyltransferase expression in pancreatic islets. Cell Physiol Biochem 2010;26: 707–716.
26 Bando M, Iwakura H, Ariyasu H, Hosoda H, Yamada G, Hosoda K, Adachi S, Nakao K, Kangawa K, Akamizu T: Transgenic overexpression of intraislet ghrelin does not affect insulin secretion or glucose metabolism in vivo. Am J Physiol Endocrinol Metab 2012;302:E403–E408.
27 Kang K, Schmahl J, Lee JM, Garcia K, Patil K, Chen A, Keene M, Murphy A, Sleeman MW: Mouse ghrelin-*O*-acyltransferase (GOAT) plays a critical role in bile acid reabsorption. FASEB J 2012;26:259–271.

Dr. Suraj Unniappan
Department of Veterinary Biomedical Sciences, Laboratory of Integrative Neuroendocrinology
Western College of Veterinary Medicine, University of Saskatchewan
52 Campus Drive, Saskatoon, SK S7N 5B4 (Canada)
E-Mail suraj.unniappan@usask.ca

Benso A, Casanueva FF, Ghigo E, Granata A (eds): The Ghrelin System.
Endocr Dev. Basel, Karger, 2013, vol 25, pp 25–40 (DOI: 10.1159/000348665)

Genetics of the Ghrelin System

Maria Gueorguiev · Márta Korbonits

Centre for Endocrinology, William Harvey Research Institute, Barts and the London School of Medicine, Queen Mary University of London, London, UK

Abstract

Ghrelin was originally identified as a growth hormone secretagogue, but later studies suggested that it plays an important role in the regulation of appetite and body weight. The implication of genetic variants of the ghrelin-ghrelin receptor axis in the determination of stature, appetite, body weight, glucose metabolism and eating disorders has been the focus of numerous small and larger studies. More recently, several studies have shown some involvement of ghrelin and growth hormone secretagogue receptor (*GHSR*) genetic variants in some cancers, or their role in the genetics of immune diseases or addictive behaviour. The overall results suggest that the effects of common genetic variants are lacking or modest, while rare sequence alteration may lead to disease status in individual patients. In this review we summarize the available data on the genetics of ghrelin axis in humans.

Members of the ghrelin axis, ghrelin, obestatin, growth hormone secretagogue receptor (GHSR) and ghrelin *O*-acyltransferase (GOAT) are candidate genes for several neuroendocrine regulatory systems regarding growth hormone release and metabolism. Ghrelin is a peptide secreted by the stomach which acts, at the level of the hypothalamic nuclei controlling food intake [1], and on the pancreas for exerting several effects on glucose homeostasis [2, 3]. Obestatin, which derives from the same precursor, preproghrelin, has, unexpectedly, been found to exert opposite effects to ghrelin on food intake in rodents, and there is no effect on growth [4]. GOAT is an enzyme which catalyses the transfer of the characteristic acyl group to the N-terminal 3rd amino acid of ghrelin. This modification is necessary for most of ghrelin's actions, although an increasing number of papers suggest important physiologic role to unacetylated ghrelin [5].

The initial linkage analyses and candidate-gene-based studies were more recently replaced by genome-wide scans involving large cohorts. These new studies were made possible by the availability of high throughput technologies which aim to increase the power for detecting the gene's effect on the studied phenotype(s). Various correlations have been detected between *GHRL*/*GHSR* genes and complex diseases/traits such as obesity, diabetes, hypertension, stature and related metabolic variables as well as cancer, but not all confirmed nor reproduced in other studies. Several biases can explain the lack of confirmation and reproducibility, the most important being differences in population selection and study design. Current evidence suggests a possible role of the *GHRL/GHSR* in susceptibility to these complex diseases and further large scale studies should be conducted to establish such associations. In addition to the effects of genetic variations, epistatic interactions involving different genes and epigenetic modifications upon environmental pressure appear to shape the phenotypes associated with complex traits diseases (obesity, diabetes mellitus and stature) as well.

Because of space limitation for this manuscript, we will focus on the role of ghrelin/growth hormone secretagogue receptor genes mainly in obesity, eating behaviour, glucose metabolism and stature, although some correlations with cardiovascular features, addictive behaviour, inflammatory diseases and cancer have been explored.

Genetic Studies in Humans

Obesity/Metabolic Syndrome

Ghrelin

The p.Leu72Met (rs696217) *GHRL* polymorphism (12.5% hetero- and 3.1% homozygotes among obese subjects; 12.5% heterozygotes among controls) showed a trend for association with earlier self-reported onset of obesity (15.6 ± 7.9 vs. 20.5 ± 10.5 years, $p = 0.09$) [6]. Further, Leu72Met was correlated with a positive family history for obesity and with born as 'large for gestational age' status [7].

A large population study of three cohorts (3,004 subjects), reported an association of Leu72Met and obesity – homozygote or heterozygote 72Met presenting the lowest BMI and lowest fat mass or less visceral fat and lower risk of metabolic disorders [8]. We and two other groups reported heterozygote Leu72Met variant to correlate with early-onset obesity among French Caucasian [9] and Italian [10], with higher ZBMI among children [9], and family history of obesity [7], although these associations could not be confirmed by others [11].

In a Japanese cohort of middle-aged and elderly men, the 72Met allele was more frequently expressed among subjects with higher BMI, thus concluding to the involvement of this single nucleotide polymorphism (SNP) in the determination of BMI [12]. Keeping in line with this observation are two other studies suggesting that the *GHRL* gene may be involved in the determination of body weight variability [13, 14]. In the first study on 112 monozygotic twin pairs, 72Met was significantly less frequent among the discordant for obesity twins than among the obese or lean-concordant twins [13]. In the Quebec Family Study, an interaction between Leu72Met (rs696217) variant and dietary fat intake and triacylglycerol concentration was found to modulate waist circumference [14]. Interestingly, in a Chinese cohort of patients with coronary artery disease, heterozygous and homozygous 72Met allele carriers

(Leu72Met andMet72Met) had a lower BMI compared to homozygous Leu72Leu carriers [15].

The prospective interventional Finnish Diabetes Prevention Study of overweight individuals with glucose intolerance or controls [16], detected that subjects with *GHRL* 72Met allele (rs696217-C) achieved more significant weight loss and waist circumference decrease by intensifying their physical activity, and that homozygous subjects for the 72Leu (rs696217-AA) had greater weight loss, independently of the intensity of physical activity [17].

The T3065C ghrelin intron variant, which is in strong linkage disequilibrium with the Leu72Met SNP, was reported to correlate with increased body weight, BMI and waist circumference, thus suggestive of a more important role of this SNP in obesity than the Leu72Met polymorphism, which did not show any association with these parameters [18].

In one of the very first reports on ghrelin, the heterozygous p.Arg51Gln (rs34911341) variant in the prepro-ghrelin was detected in 6.3%, exclusively among obese female unrelated subjects with lower weight compared to the wild type [6].

Although the Gln90Leu (rs4684677) prepro-ghrelin/obestatin variant was more frequently identified in a group of extremely obese subjects compared to normal weight, the analysis could not show a link for any features of obesity [11]. In a family-based case-control study, we found a correlation between ghrelin polymorphism Gln90Leu (rs4684677) with obesity, but confirmation was not obtained following correction for multiple testing and replication in a German genomewide association study [19]. Thus, although minor effects of common ghrelin SNPs may influence several phenotypic traits linked to obesity, they do not provide a major contribution to polygenic obesity.

In the absence of a significant correlation between 11 SNPs genotypes (located in the 5′ flanking region of ghrelin gene), and fasting plasma ghrelin concentrations in the total OPERA population (Oulu Project Elucidating Risk for Atherosclerosis cohort), the SNP-501A>C (rs26802) showed borderline association with lower BMI and waist circumference, but showed a differential genotype distribution among subjects with highest versus lowest plasma ghrelin levels [20], thus a possible involvement in the determination of BMI and waist circumference should be confirmed by larger studies.

In this context, the -501C ghrelin allele was correlated with higher postprandial levels of the anorexigenic PYY hormone [21], thus supporting a role in the regulation of BMI.

A large-scale case-control European study (EPIC – European Prospective Investigation into Cancer and Nutrition including 1359 women with breast cancer and 2389 matched controls) found a significant correlation between several *GHRL* SNPs (rs171336, rs171407, rs27498, rs3755777) and obesity, BMI, but because of a false-positive report probability <25%, it is necessary to carefully interpret such results [22].

Interestingly, a study identified a rare ghrelin promoter variant, –151T>C, which completely cosegregated with obesity in a Danish family, and incompletely cosegregated in a Czech family, likely due to an incomplete penetrance of this variant [23], thus suggesting a major involvement of this variant in obesity. However, this ghrelin variant did not correlate with a Three Factor Eating Questionnaire neither was it detected in the rest of the cohort studied [23].

Growth Hormone Secretagogue Receptor

The prospective interventional Finnish Diabetes Prevention Study including overweight subjects with glucose intolerance and controls, reported strong linkage disequilibrium between two *GHSR* variants, rs490683 and rs509035 [20]. In a later study deriving from the same population, individuals (with glucose intolerance and controls) carrying the homozygous rs490683-CC genotype achieved greater weight loss submitted to exercising during the 3-year study duration whilst those carrying rs9819506-G allele presented with higher weight [24].

Two *GHSR* promoter polymorphisms (rs490683 and rs9819506) have shown significant association with weight loss in subjects of mixed European ancestry who have previously undergone a Roux-en-Y gastric bypass surgery [25]. More specifically, individuals homozygous for the rs490683-CC obtained 5% greater weight loss in the first 30 post-operative months compared to the others [25]. The authors speculated that decreasing the *GHSR* activity/signalling could decrease appetite and weight loss as a counterbalance for the ghrelin overproduction following this type of surgery based on the reduction of *GHSR* promoter activity by 20% for rs490683-CC genotype observed in vitro [25].

In our Ely population-based study for investigating the aetiology and pathogenesis of type 2 diabetes and related metabolic disorders in adults, we found a borderline association between *GHSR* c.171T>C (p.Gly57Gly, rs495225) and BMI, but this association was not significant after correction and did not replicate these results in other cohorts [26].

We also detected a link between *GHSR* SNP rs572169 and obesity in our family-based case-control study, but further confirmation following correction for multiple testing and replication was not observed [19]. We therefore concluded that this variant was not directly connected to polygenic obesity despite possibly affecting to a limited point, several phenotypic traits linked to obesity. In addition, an association study failed to detect significant link between several *GHRS* variants, at the single or haplotype level, with obesity in a large cohort of 15,854 unrelated subjects [22]. These data support our own conclusion that common SNPs of the *GHSR* do not have a major role in the development of polygenic obesity [19]. A smaller population-based Australian retrospective longitudinal study of 1,362 children with idiopathic short stature (ISS) or growth hormone deficiency (GHD), followed from birth to 10 years of age, did not find any association for five ghrelin receptor variants with weight or BMI [27], repeating earlier observations.

The correlation of *GHSR* 477G>A allele (rs572169) with higher postprandial plasma levels of the anorexigenic PYY hormone suggests a contributory role in the regulation of BMI [21].

In the EPIC study – the *GHSR* SNP (rs572169) correlated significantly with obesity and BMI, but the interpretation of these results should be tempered (false-positive report probability <25%) [21].

However, one rare mutation, c.611C>A (p.Ala204Glu, rs121917883), was identified in an obese subject and a second rare mutation, c.837C>A (p.Phe279Leu, SNP002901686) was detected in a child with short normal stature and his mother affected with obesity and short stature [28].

Eating Behaviour

Bulimia nervosa

Ghrelin

Despite the lack of implication of ghrelin SNPs in anorexia, bulimia or binge-eating behaviour in some studies [29–31], others have detected associations. *GHSR* polymorphism c.171C>T (Gly57Gly, rs495225) and ghrelin variants Leu72Met (rs696217) and rs2075356, individually or as a haplotype, were correlated with bulimia and binge-eating, respectively, in Japanese cohorts (including also non-obese subjects). The Leu72Met variant was also linked with higher hunger scores among subjects of the Old Order Amish [32]. The Leu72Met and the 3056T>C polymorphisms of the prepro-ghrelin gene were associated with susceptibility to bulimia nervosa purging type [33].

Growth Hormone Secretagogue Receptor

We observed an association between *GHSR* polymorphisms rs2232169 (Leu49Leu, C447G) and 'overeating' in Caucasian obese individuals [19]. However, this observation was not confirmed after correction for multiple testing [19], thus limiting the effects of this variant in obesity whilst still potentially modulating the eating phenotype.

GHSR SNPs have been involved in bulimia nervosa as well. Thus, 171C>T (Gly57Gly, rs495225) genotype was detected more frequently in Japanese patients with this disorder and not in controls [34].

There was a correlation between dietary restraint and disinhibition, as well as perceived hunger with the *GHSR* 477G>A (rs572169) polymorphism [21].

Anorexia Nervosa

Ghrelin

A French familial study detected a preferential transmission (transmission disequilibrium) of Leu72Met and binge eating/purging among 114 probands affected with anorexia nervosa and their parents [35]. The Gln90/Leu72 haplotype (rs4684677/rs696217) of the prepro-ghrelin/obestatin gene was transmitted preferentially among subjects with anorexia nervosa [35]. These data support the observation that these ghrelin SNPs confer susceptibility to anorexia nervosa.

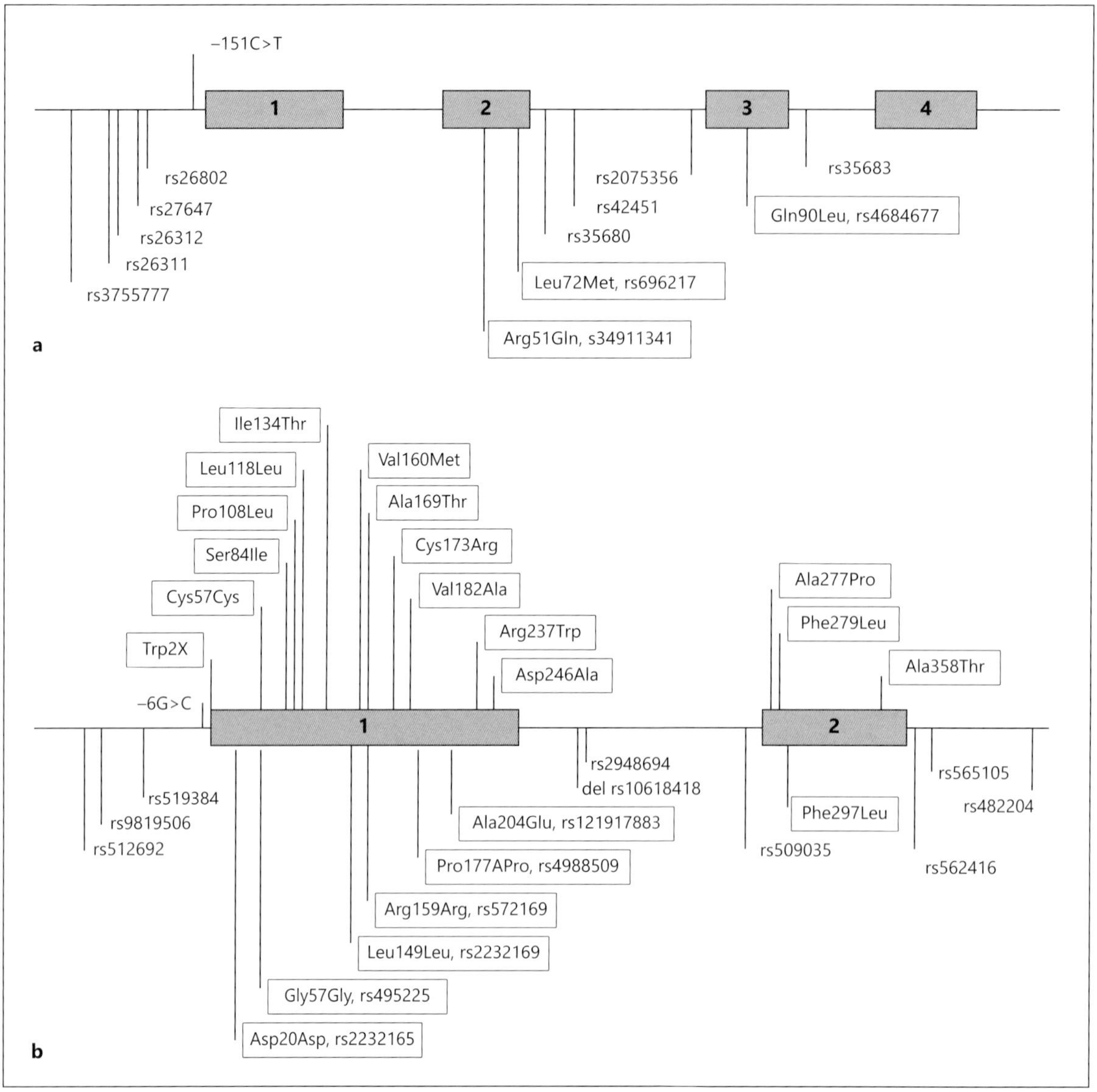

Fig. 1. a Prepro-ghrelin (chromosome 3p25.3). Ghrelin gene *(GHRL)* common polymorphisms (bottom) and rare variants (top) reported in the literature are shown. **b** GHSR (chromosome 3q26.31). Growth hormone secretagogue receptor gene *(GHSR)* common polymorphisms (bottom) and rare variants (top) reported in the literature are shown.

GOAT

A German group assessed the genetic variance of *GOAT* (a 6 tagging SNPs haplotype) and feeding behaviour. Among two populations – an obese cohort (543 individuals) and healthy and underweight controls (612 subjects) *GOAT* was found to be involved in anorexia nervosa on the basis of association of a SNP (rs10096079) with anorexia nervosa [36].

Metabolism

Glucose/Diabetes

Ghrelin

We reported a correlation between ghrelin Leu72Met (rs696217) heterozygote variant with reduced insulin secretion during the first phase of an oral glucose tolerance test (OGTT) among obese French Caucasian children, suggesting the existence of alterations in insulin and glucose metabolism [9]. In support of this conclusion, subjects carrying Leu72Leu were found to be at lower risk for the development of type 2 diabetes [37]. Increased fasting glucose was associated with the Leu72Met ghrelin variant in the Old Order Amish [38]. In an Italian case-control cohort (overweight/obese subjects and healthy matched controls), both 72Leu and 72Met alleles were shown to exert a co-dominant effect on the phenotype that translated by an association between the increasing number of 72Met alleles and lower fasting insulin levels and HOMA-IR [38]. This SNP was found to be in strong linkage disequilibrium with a ghrelin promoter SNP (–604C>T, rs27647), which had a similar trend for reducing insulin and HOMA-IR, individually or as a haplotype [38].

We detected an association between ghrelin polymorphism –604A>G (rs27647) and insulin levels at 2 h after an OGTT in Caucasian obese individuals [19]. However, this observation was not confirmed after correction for multiple testing [19], thus limiting the effects of this variant in obesity whilst conserving a potential impact on insulin secretion.

Contradictory observations were reported for the 72Met variant (rs696217) being associated with decreased risk for type 2 diabetes mellitus in a Caucasian case-control study [39]. A meta-analysis of several different studies has also concluded to an association between 72Met variant and a reduced risk of type 2 diabetes mellitus among Caucasians [40]. Other studies – one on monozygotic twin pairs and the Quebec Family Study – showed that Leu72Met (rs696217) variant was not associated with type 2 diabetes mellitus nor with fasting glycaemia nor insulinaemia [13, 14]. We also did not find a correlation for *GHRL* and *GHSR* polymorphisms and type 2 diabetes mellitus [41].

Although ghrelin Arg51Gln variant (rs34911341), which represents a proteolytic site for cleavage that allows generating mature ghrelin, was considered to represent a risk factor for type 2 diabetes in middle-aged subjects [42], others have failed to find any association between ghrelin gene polymorphisms and type 2 diabetes [43]. The Arg51 was also found to protect against metabolic syndrome [44].

In addition, the *GHRL* Arg51Gly (rs34911341) SNP was found to be protective against gestational diabetes mellitus in a small cohort of Brazilian pregnant women by reducing 5 times the risk for this disease [45].

Growth Hormone Secretagogue Receptor

Vartiainen et al. [46] reported a correlation between *GHSR* 171C>T (rs495225) and 477C>A (rs572169) variants and the values of the area under the insulin curve values during an OGTT.

From the Finnish Diabetes Prevention Study of overweight subjects either with impaired glucose tolerance or controls, individuals from the entire cohort and the control group harbouring homozygous rs490683-CC or rs509035-TT genotypes from the *GHSR* gene had the lowest 2-hour glucose and insulin levels all along the duration of the study [47].

Lipid Metabolism

Ghrelin

A correlation between the Leu72Met polymorphism and lower plasma lipoprotein(a) levels has been reported in type 2 diabetic patients [48]. In the Old Order Amish cohort, low HDL and high triglyceride plasma levels were correlated with Leu72Met SNP [32]. Patients carrying 72Met had lower total cholesterol in patients with diabetic nephropathy and renal dysfunction [49]. However, other studies could not find any association of this SNP with serum lipid profile among patients with type 2 diabetes mellitus or metabolic syndrome [16, 61].

Two ghrelin polymorphisms, –1062G>C and T3065C (in strong linkage disequilibrium with Leu72Met, rs696217), were found to correlate with lower plasma HDL cholesterol levels among non-diabetic Korean subjects and Japanese women [43, 17].

Growth Hormone Secretagogue Receptor

In a Finish cohort (OPERA), *GHSR* 477G>A SNP (rs572169) and plasma LDL and VLDL levels correlated [46].

Stature

Ghrelin

Ghrelin rs696217 (Leu72Met) variant was shown to correlate with higher IGF-1 levels in Black subjects in the Heritage Family Study [8] and in obese/overweight Italian children [7]. Ghrelin rs375577 polymorphism showed a positive correlation with circulating IGF-1 levels, and rs2075356 had a borderline significant correlation with IGFBP-3 levels for homozygous carriers of the minor alleles in the EPIC breast cancer risk population [22].

However, ghrelin polymorphisms were not associated with either idiopathic short stature (n = 81) or growth hormone deficiency (n = 117) among Chinese children [47]. Our study of familial association testing on French obese tall children and controls corroborated this observation [48]. We did not find any correlation between ghrelin SNPs and stature, which is in favour of the assertion that common *ghrelin* genetic variants are not implicated in the determination of height variation in the French population [48].

In the EPIC Study a significant correlation between *GHRL* SNPs (rs171336, rs171407, rs27498, rs3755777) and height was found [22]. However, these results need careful interpretation as the false-positive report probability was <25% [22].

We refined a previous GWAS analysis (which has shown linkage for chromosome 3p26 locus, a locus close to the ghrelin gene, with height (lod score 3.17)) by screening

Table 1. Associations between ghrelin and GHSR genetic variants reported in the literature

a Associations of ghrelin and GHSR polymorphisms with obesity

Gene	SNP/mutation	Association	Study ref.
Ghrelin	−501A>C, rs26802	Alleles A: trend for association with higher BMI and waist circumference	[20]
		Allele C: correlation with higher post prandial plasma PYY levels	[15]
	−151T>C	Complete co-segregation with obesity in a Danish family, incomplete co-segregation in a Czeh family	[21]
	rs3755777	Homozygotes minor allele: increased risk for obesity (careful FFRP <25%)	[22]
		Association with obesity (careful FFRP <25%)	
	rs27498	Association with obesity (careful FFRP <25%)	[22]
	Arg51Gln, rs34911341	Heterozygous, prevalence 6.3% among obese female with lower weight	[6]
	Leu72Met, rs696217	Prevalence 12.5 and 3.5% hetero- and homozygous among obese	[6]
		Trends for association with earlier onset of obesity	[6]
		Correlation with positive family history for obesity and born large for gestational age	[7]
		Association with obesity, lowest BMI, and lowest fat mass or less visceral fat and lower risk of metabolic disorders	[8]
		Heterozygous SNP: correlation with early-onset obesity	[9]
		72Met: higher expression among middle-aged and elderly Japanese men	[12]
		72Met: lower prevalence among monozygotic twins	[13]
		Interaction between Leu72Met and dietary fat intake and triacylglycerol concentration, causing modulation of waist circumference	[14]
		72Met: greater weight loss and waist circumference by intensifying exercice	[16]
		homozygous 72Leu greater weight loss independent of physical activity	[17]
		Leu72Met & Met72Met: associated with lower BMI	[15]
	Gln90Leu, rs4684677	Prevalent in extremely obese subjects	[11]
	3065T>C	Strong linkage disequilibrium with Leu72Met	[33]
		Correlation with increased body weight, BMI and waist circumference	
	rs171336	Association with obesity, BMI (careful FFRP<25%)	[22]
	rs171407	Association with obesity, BMI (careful FFRP<25%)	[22]
GHSR	rs490683	Homozygous CC: association with greater weight loss among subjects with glucose intolerance and controls during exercising program	[46]
		5% greater weight loss postoperative (Roux-en-Y gastric bypass)	[25]
	rs509035	G allele: association with higher weight	[46]
	Arg159Arg, rs572169	Association with obesity (careful FFRP<25%)	[22]
	rs9819506	Weight loss post-operative (Roux-en-Y gastric bypass)	[25]

b Associations of ghrelin and GHSR polymorphisms with eating behaviour

Gene	SNP/mutation	Association	Study ref.
Ghrelin	Leu72Met, rsrs696217	Association with higher hunger scores	[32]
		Association with BN-P bulimia nervosa purging type	[33]
		Preferential transmission of Leu72Met and binge eating/purging among patients with anorexia nervosa (AN)	[35]
	Gln90Leu72 haplotype	Preferential transmission among AN subjects	[35]
	3056T>C, rs2075356	Association with BN-P bulimia nervosa purging type TT genotype: association with higher probability and rate for recovery of normal weight	[33]
	72Met-3056C haplotype	Increased frequency among patinets with BN-P	[33]

Table 1. Continued

Gene	SNP/mutation	Association	Study ref.
GHSR	171T>C, rs495225	CC genotype: higher frequency among subjects with BN, risk factor for BN	[34]
	Arg159Arg, rs2232169	Correlation with dietary restraint and disinhibition, and perceived hunger	[21]
GOAT	rs100096079	Association with AN	[36]

c Associations of ghrelin and GHSR polymorphisms with glucose metabolism

Gene	SNP/mutation	Association	Study ref.
Ghrelin	–604C>T, rs27647	Trend for association with lower insulin and HOMA-IR	[38]
	Arg51Gln, rs34911341	Risk factor for T2DM in middle-aged subjects	[42]
		Arg51 allele: protective role against metabolic syndrome	[32]
		Arg51Gln: protective role against gestational diabetes	[44]
	Leu72Met, rs696217	Heterozygote: correlation with reduced insulin secretion during the first phase of OGTT in obese children	[9]
		Heterozygote: association with increased fasting glucose	[32]
		Leu72Leu: lower risk for development of type 2 diabetes mellitus	[37]
		72Met: association with lower fasting insulin levels and HOMA-IR	[53]
		72Met: association with reduced risk for DMT2	[39]
GHSR	171C>T, rs495225	Correlation with the area under the insulin curve values during an OGTT	[45]
	Arg159Arg, rs572169	Correlation with the area under the insulin curve values during an OGTT	[45]
	rs490683_CC	Association with the lowest 2-h glucose and insulin levels	[46]
	rs509035-TT	Association with the lowest 2-h glucose and insulin levels	[46]

d Associations of ghrelin and GHSR polymorphisms with stature

Gene	SNP/mutation	Association	Study ref.
Ghrelin	rs171336, rs171407, rs27498, rs3755777	Association with height (caution in interpreting as FPRP < 25%)	[22]
GHSR	rs572169	Association with height (caution in interpreting as FPRP < 25%)	[22]
		Site associated for height in humans	[51]
	rs482204	TT genotype associated with greater stature at all ages	[27]
	rs562416	TT genotype correlated with tall stature at age 3, 8, and 10 years	
	Ala204Glu (SNP0029001685)	Segregated with idiopathic short stature in two unrelated families 1 obese subject	[28]
		Associated with idiopathic short stature and with isolated GH deficiency respectively in two unrelated Moroccan families	[52]
	837C>A (Phe279Leu, SNP002901686)	Detected in an individual with short stature and in a proband	[28]
	c.6G>A, W2X and c.709A>T, R237W	Heterozygous associated with GH deficiency, hypoglycaemia and ketosis	[54]
	ΔQ36 (c.106-108 del CAG)	Detected in 3 patients from 3 different families with idiopathic short stature and in one control	[55]
	P108L (c.323C>T)	Detected in 1 patient with idiopathic short stature	
	C173R (c.17T>C)	Detected in 1 patient with idiopathic short stature	
	D264A (c.737A>C)	Detected in 3 patients from a family with idiopathic short stature Cumulative frequency of mutations higher in patients with ISS than controls (4.72 vs. 0.53%, p 0 0.019, OR 9.28, 95% CI 1.10–78.0)	

Table 1. Continued

Gene	SNP/mutation	Association	Study ref.
	c.-6G>C	Found in a patient with CDGP	[56]
	c.215G>T (Ser84Ile)	Mutation found in a patient with CDGP and in two normal siblings	
	c.505G>A (Ala169Thr)	Found in a patient with CDGP	
	c.545T>C (Val182Ala)	Mutation found in a patient, a sibling and her father, all with CDGP	
	c.1072G>A (Ala358Thr)	Found in a patient with CDGP Cumulative mutations frequency higher in the CDGP than in children with ISS and in the control group	

for association between additional microsatellite markers around GHRL that we genotyped in the Warren 2 UK cohort, and adult stature [49]. In the absence of such association, we concluded that ghrelin variants could not explain the observed variation in adult height [49].

Growth Hormone Secretagogue Receptor

The *GHSR* 171CC variant (Gly57Gly, rs495225) correlated with lower IGF-BP1 levels and higher area under the insulin curve in an oral glucose tolerance test, findings consistent with type 2 diabetes and obesity, or insulin resistance [45]. We could not confirm a positive association for *GHSR* variant 477G>A (Arg159Arg, rs572169) with IGF-1 levels, after correction and replication [50].

Our study of familial association testing on French obese children and controls corroborated this observation [48]. We found that the absence of a 2-bp deletion in the *GHSR* gene or a heterozygous status was more frequently encountered among tall obese children; however, this association was not confirmed after correction for multiple testing [48]. There was also no evidence for interaction between different variants of these genes that could suggest an implication in the determination of stature [48]. Therefore, we concluded that common *GHSR* polymorphisms do not play a major role in determining height variation in the French population [48].

In addition, we studied 3 larger UK cohorts: two cohorts with adults – the Medical Research Council Ely Study (Caucasian population for the study of the aetiology and pathogenesis of type 2 diabetes and related metabolic disorders, n = 811, and EPIC, n = 4,996 healthy subjects); one cohort with children (ALSPAC, Avon Longitudinal Study of Parents and Children, n = 843) [50]. We observed only a weak inverse association between *GHSR* 477G>A (rs2232169) minor allele and height, which was not significant after correction and replication [50].

In the EPIC Study, a significant correlation between *GHSR* SNP (rs572169) and height was found [28]. Again, it is important to stress that the interpretation of these results needs caution as the false-positive report probability was <25% [22].

Recently, two *GHSR* polymorphisms were found to be associated with stature throughout childhood in a population-based Australian retrospective longitudinal study including 1,362 children from birth to 10 years of age [27]: both rs482204 TT and rs562416 TT genotypes correlated significantly with higher/taller stature at different ages of observation (3, 8 and 10 years).

However, a larger cohort of 180,000 successfully identified the *GHSR* SNP rs572169 as a site for associated height in humans and confirmed by a family-based study on 7,336 subjects [51]. It is very likely that because of the very low magnitude of the effects of common gene variants to contribute to human height/stature, only very large studies have the power to detect it.

Wang et al. [28] discovered a rare mutation within *GHSR*, Phe279Leu (SNP002901686), in one child with short normal stature whose mother has both short stature and obesity. In addition, Ala204Glu (rs121917883) missense mutation, causing loss of constitutive activity of *GHSR*, has been found to segregate with short stature within two unrelated families [52], and has been initially described by Wang et al. [28] in an obese carrier. Phenotypically, the only patient homozygous for this mutation had a presentation with ISS, while heterozygous members had either ISS or isolated GHD [52]. Homozygous/heterozygous subjects of one of the families were either obese or with a slight tendency to be overweight as opposed to the heterozygous individuals from the other family presenting rather with a normal weight or with a tendency to be lean [53]. This Ala204Glu variant resulted in a GHSR1A peptide with decreased cell-surface expression and decreased binding of its ligand, ghrelin, but without altering the affinity for ghrelin [52]. Subsequently, the same group identified two other rare missense mutations within the ghrelin receptor (c.6G>A, p.Trp2* and c.709A>T, p.Arg237Trp) causing growth hormone deficiency associated with hypoglycaemia and ketosis, abdominal pain and vomiting, and low BMI in a subject compound heterozygote for these two mutations in the GHSR receptor [54]. Each parent carried one of the mutations, either p.Trp2* by his healthy father, or the p. Arg237Trp by his healthy mother [93]. In vitro studies have shown that the p. Arg237Trp mutation leads to partial loss of constitutive activity of GHSR, and both, Val160Met and Phe279Leu mutations also showed a significant reduction in basal and constitutive activity [54].

Seven rare *GHSR* variants were detected among a cohort of unrelated Japanese individuals with ISS (n = 113) or with GHD (n = 14) compared to controls [55]. Among these variants were a 3-bp in-frame heterozygous deletion ΔQ36 (detected in 3 patients and one control), 4 missense heterozygous substitutions – Pro108Leu, Cys173Arg, Asp246Ala, Ala277Pro (the first three detected each in one patient, whilst the later was found in one patient and 3 controls), and 3 synonymous changes – Cys57Cys, Leu118Leu and Arg159Arg [55]. Prediction analyses and/or functional studies showed that all four novel mutations Pro108Leu, Cys173Arg, ΔQ36 and Asp246Ala resulted in decreased constitutive activity of the receptor to various degrees, or altered interaction [55]. The significantly higher cumulative incidence of these mutations among the affected patients compared to the controls, and the functional defects suggest that GHSR mutations contribute to short stature [55].

A Brazilian study reported five heterozygous mutations (c.–6G>C, c.215G>T (p. Ser84Ile), c.505G>A (p.Ala169Thr), c.545T>C (p.Val182Ala), c.1072G>A (p.Ala358Thr)) in the *GHSR* gene among children with constitutional delay of growth and puberty, a condition considered as a subtype of ISS [56]. For two of the mutations in particular, the corresponding family genotypes and phenotypes revealed that a patient with constitutional delay of growth and puberty (CDGP) and two normal siblings were harbouring the variant Ser84Ile; the other gene variant, Val182Ala, was detected in a patient, a sibling and her father, all with CDGP [56]. Ser84Ile missense mutation was shown to induce a decrease in ghrelin potency/efficacy, and both mutations showed decreased basal activity vs. wild type [56]. Interestingly, both mutations carriers identified at the age of 13 with height SDS of –2.4 and –2.3, progressed normally through puberty and did not require any therapy to reach normal adult height (height SDS –0.7 and –1.4) [56]. The cumulative mutations frequency was higher in the CDGP group than in children with ISS and in the control group, which is in support of a role of *GHSR* gene in CDGP [56].

Conclusions

Metabolic variables and height are determined by an essentially polygenic manner. Common *GHRL* and *GHSR* variants do not appear to be prominently involved in the determination of these traits, although their modest effect may modulate a particular phenotype. One of the largest genetic studies suggests that among many other genes, *GHSR* is involved in the determination of height. In addition to the intricate interaction between SNPs within the same gene or between different genes (such as linkage disequilibrium and epistatic interactions), epigenetic changes could also influence complex traits.

References

1 Nakazato M, Murakami N, Date Y, Kojima M, Matsuo H, Kangawa K, Matsukura S: A role for ghrelin in the central regulation of feeding. Nature 2001;409:194–198.

2 Broglio F, Arvat E, Benso A, Gottero C, Muccioli G, Papotti M, van der Lely AJ, Deghenghi R, Ghigo E: Ghrelin, a natural GH secretagogue produced by the stomach, induces hyperglycemia and reduces insulin secretion in humans. J Clin Endocrinol Metab 2001; 86:5083–5086.

3 Kojima M, Hosoda H, Date Y, Nakazato M, Matsuo H, Kangawa K: Ghrelin is a growth-hormone-releasing acylated peptide from stomach. Nature 1999;402:656–660.

4 Zhang JV, Ren PG, Avsian-Kretchmer O, Luo CW, Rauch R, Klein C, Hsueh AJ: Obestatin, a peptide encoded by the ghrelin gene, opposes ghrelin's effects on food intake. Science 2005;310:996–999.

5 Benso A, St-Pierre DH, Prodam F, Gramaglia E, Granata R, van der Lely AJ, Ghigo E, Broglio F: Metabolic effects of overnight continuous infusion of unacylated ghrelin in humans. Eur J Endocrinol. 2012;166:911–916.
6 Ukkola O, Ravussen E, Jacobson P, et al: Rapid communications: mutations in the ghrelin/preproghrelin gene associated with obesity in humans. J Clin Endocrinol Metab 2001;86:3996–3999.
7 Vivenza D, Rapa A, Castellino N, et al: Ghrelin gene polymorphisms and ghrelin, insulin, IGF-1, leptin and anthropometric data in children and adolescents. Eur J Endocrinol 2004;151:127–133.
8 Ukkola O, Ravussen E, Jacobson P, et al: Role of ghrelin polymorphisms in obesity based on three different studies. Obes Res 2002;10:782–791.
9 Korbonits M, Gueorguiev M, O'Grady E, Lecoeur C, Swan DC, Mein CA, Weill J, Grossman AB, Froguel P: A variation in the ghrelin gene increases weight and decreases insulin secretion in tall, obese children. J Clin Endocrinol Metab 2002;87:4005–4008.
10 Miraglia DG, Santoro N, Cirillo G, et al: Molecular screening of the ghrelin gene in Italian obese children: the Leu72Met variant is associated with an earlier onset of obesity. Int J Obes Relat Metab Disord 2002;28:447–450.
11 Hinney A, Hoch A, Geller F, et al: Ghrelin gene: identification of missense variants and a frameshift mutation in extremely obese children and adolescents and healthy normal weight students. J Clin Endocrinol Metab 2002;87:2716–2719.
12 Kuzuya M, Ando F, Iguchi A, Shimokata H: Preproghrelin Leu72Met variant contributes to overweight in middle-aged men of a Japanese large cohort. Int J Obes (Lond) 2006;30:1609–1614.
13 Leskelä P, Ukkola O, Vartiainen J, Rönnemaa T, Kaprio J, Bouchard C, Kesäniemi YA: Fasting plasma total ghrelin concentrations in monozygotic twins discordant for obesity. Metabolism 2009;58:174–179.
14 Robitaille J, Pérusse L, Bouchard C, Vohl MC: Genes, fat intake, and cardiovascular disease risk factors in the Quebec Family Study. Obesity (Silver Spring) 2007;15:2336–2347.
15 Tang NP, Wang LS, Yang L, Gu HJ, Zhu HJ, Zhou B, Sun QM, Cong RH, Wang B: Preproghrelin Leu72Met polymorphism in Chinese subjects with coronary artery disease and controls. Clin Chim Acta 2008;387:42–47.
16 Tuomilehto J, Lindström J, Eriksson JG, Valle TT, Hämäläinen H, Ilanne-Parikka P, Keinänen-Kiukaanniemi S, Laakso M, Louheranta A, Rastas M, Salminen V, Uusitupa M, Finnish Diabetes Prevention Study Group: Prevention of type 2 diabetes mellitus by changes in life style among subjects with impaired glucose tolerance. N Engl J Med 2001;344:1343–1350.
17 Kilpeläinen TO, Lakka TA, Laaksonen DE, Mager U, Salopuro T, Kubaszek A, Todorova B, Laukkanen O, Lindström J, Eriksson JG, Hämäläinen H, Aunola S, Ilanne-Parikka P, Keinänen-Kiukaanniemi S, Tuomilehto J, Laakso M, Uusitupa M, Finnish Diabetes Prevention Study Group: Interaction of single nucleotide polymorphisms in ADRB2, ADRB3, TNF, IL6, IGF1R, LIPC, LEPR, and GHRL with physical activity on the risk of type 2 diabetes mellitus and changes in characteristics of the metabolic syndrome: The Finnish Diabetes Prevention Study. Metabolism 2008;57:428–436.
18 Ando T, Ichimaru Y, Konjiki F, Shoji M, Komaki G: Variations in the preproghrelin gene correlate with higher body mass index, fat mass, and body dissatisfaction in young Japanese women. Am J Clin Nutr 2007;86:25–32.
19 Gueorguiev M, Lecoeur C, Meyre D, Benzinou M, Mein CA, Hinney A, Vatin V, Weill J, Heude B, Hebebrand J, Grossman AB, Korbonits M, Froguel P: Association studies on ghrelin and ghrelin receptor gene polymorphisms with obesity. Obesity (Silver Spring) 2009;17:745–754.
20 Vartiainen J, Kesaniemi YA, Ukkola O: Sequencing analysis of ghrelin gene 5′ flanking region: relations between the sequence variants, fasting plasma total ghrelin concentrations, and body mass index. Metabolism 2006;55:1420–1425.
21 den Hoed M, Smeets AJ, Veldhorst MA, Nieuwenhuizen AG, Bouwman FG, Heidema AG, Mariman EC, Westerterp-Plantenga MS, Westerterp KR: SNP analyses of postprandial responses in (an)orexigenic hormones and feelings of hunger reveal long-term physiological adaptations to facilitate homeostasis. Int J Obes (Lond) 2008;32:1790–1798.
22 Dossus L, McKay JD, Canzian F, et al: Polymorphisms of genes coding for ghrelin and its receptor in relation to anthropometry, circulating levels of IGF-I and IGFBP-3, and breast cancer risk: a case-control study nested within the European Prospective Investigation into Cancer and Nutrition (EPIC). Carcinogenesis 2008;29:1360–1366.
23 Gjesing AP, Larsen LH, Torekov SS, Hainerová IA, Kapur R, Johansen A, Albrechtsen A, Boj S, Holst B, Harper A, Urhammer SA, Borch-Johnsen K, Pisinger C, Echwald SM, Eiberg H, Astrup A, Lebl J, Ferrer J, Schwartz TW, Hansen T, Pedersen O: Family and population-based studies on variation within the ghrelin receptor locus in relation to measures of obesity. PlosOne 2010;5:e10084.
24 Mager U, Kolehmainen M, Lindström J, Eriksson JG, Valle TT, Hämäläinen H, Ilanne-Parikka P, Keinänen-Kiukaanniemi S, Tuomilehto JO, Pulkkinen L, Uusitupa MI, Finnish Diabetes Prevention Study Group: Association between ghrelin gene variations and blood pressure in subjects with impaired glucose tolerance. Am J Hypertens 2006;19:920–926.

25 Matzko ME, Argyropoulos G, Wood GC, Chu X, McCarter RJ, Still CD, Gerhard GS: Association of ghrelin receptor promoter polymorphisms with weight loss following Roux-en-Y gastric bypass surgery. Obes Surg 2012;22:783–790.
26 Garcia EA, Heude B, Petry CJ, Gueorguiev M, Hassan-Smith ZK, Spanou A, Ring SM, Dunger DB, Wareham N, Sandhu MS, Ong KK, Korbonits M: Ghrelin receptor gene polymorphisms and body size in children and adults. J Clin Endocrinol Metab. 2008;93:4158–4161.
27 Riedl S, Hughes I, Harris M, Leong GM, Beilby J, Sly P, Choong CS: Growth hormone secretagogue receptor (GHSR) gene polymorphishms are associated with stature throughout pregnancy. Eur J Endocrinol 2012;166:1079–1085.
28 Wang HJ, Geller F, Dempfle A Schäuble N, Friedel S, Lichtner P, Fontenla-Horro F, Wudy S, Hagemann S, Gortner L, Huse K, Remschmidt H, Bettecken T, Meitinger T, Schäfer H, Hebebrand J, Hinney A: Ghrelin receptor gene: identification of several sequence variants in extremely obese children and adolescents, healthy normal-weight and underweight students, and children with short normal stature. J Clin Endocrinol Metab 2004;89:157–162.
29 Cellini E, Nacmias B, Brecelj-Anderluh M, et al: Case-control and combined family trios analysis of three polymorphisms in the ghrelin gene in European patients with anorexia and bulimia nervosa. Psychiatr Genet 2006;16:51–52.
30 Monteleone P, Tortorella A, Castaldo E, Di Filippo C, Maj M: No association of the Arg51Gln and Leu72Met polymorphisms of the ghrelin gene with anorexia nervosa or bulimia nervosa. Neurosci Lett 2006;398:325–327.
31 Kindler J, Bailer U, de Zwaan M, Fuchs K, Leisch F, Grün B, Strnad A, Stojanovic M, Windisch J, Lennkh-Wolfsberg C, El-Giamal N, Sieghart W, Kasper S, Aschauer H: No association of the neuropeptide Y (Leu7Pro) and ghrelin gene (Arg51Gln, Leu72Met, Gln90Leu) single nucleotide polymorphisms with eating disorders. Nord J Psychiatry 2011;65:203–207.
32 Steinle NI, Pollin TI, O'Connell JR, Mitchell BD, Shuldiner AR: Variants in the ghrelin gene are associated with metabolic syndrome in the Old Order Amish. J Clin Endocrinol Metab 2005;90:6672–6677.
33 Ando T, Komaki G, Naruo T, et al: Possible role of preproghrelin gene polymorphisms in susceptibility to bulimia nervosa. Am J Med Genet B Neuropsychiatr Genet 2006;141B:929–934.
34 Miyasaka K, Hosoya H, Sekime A, Ohta M, Amono H, Matsushita S, Suzuki K, Higuchi S, Funakoshi A: Association of ghrelin receptor gene polymorphism with Bulimia nervosa in a Japanese population. J Neural Transm 2006;113:1279–1285.
35 Dardennes RM, Zizzari P, TolleV, Foulon C, Kipman A, Romo L, Iancu-Gontard D, Boni C, Sinet PM, Thérèse Bluet M, Estour B, Mouren MC, Guelfi JD, Rouillon F, Gorwood P, Epelbaum J: Famiy trios analysis of common polymorphisms in the obestatin/ghrelin, BDNF and AGRP genes in patients with anorexia nervosa: association with subtype, body mass index, severity and age of onset. Psychoneuroendocrinology 2007;32:106–113.
36 Müller TD, Tschöp MH, Jarick I, Ehrlich S, Scherag S, Herpertz-Dahlmann B, Zipfel S, Herzog W, de Zwaan M, Burghardt R, Fleischhaker C, Klampfl K, Wewetzer C, Herpertz S, Zeeck A, Tagay S, Burgmer M, Pfluger PT, Scherag A, Hebebrand J, Hinney A: Genetic variation of the ghrelin activator gene ghrelin O-acyltransferase (GOAT) is associated with anorexia nervosa. J Psychiatr Res 2011;45:706–711.
37 Mager U, Lindi V, Lindstrom J Eriksson JG, Valle TT, Hämäläinen H, Ilanne-Parikka P, Keinänen-Kiukaanniemi S, Tuomilehto J, Laakso M, Pulkkinen L, Uusitupa M, Finnish Diabetes Prevention Study Group: Association of the Leu72Met polymorphism of the ghrelin gene with the risk of type 2 diabetes in subjects with impaired glucose tolerance in the Finnish Diabetes Prevention Study. Diabet Med 2006;23:685–689.
38 Zavarella S, Petrone A, Zampetti S, Gueorguiev M, Spoletini M, Mein CA, Leto G, Korbonits M, Buzzetti R: A new variation in the promoter region, the –604C>T, and the Leu72Met polymorphism of the ghrelin gene are associated with protection to insulin resistance. Int J Obes 2008;32:663–668.
39 Berthold HK, Giannakidou E, Krone W, Mantzoros CS, Gouni-Berthold I: The Leu72Met polymorphism of the ghrelin gene is associated with decreased risk for type 2 diabetes. Clin Chim Acta 2009;399:112–116.
40 Liao N, Xie ZK, Huang J, Xie ZF: Association between the ghrelin Leu72Met polymorphism and type 2 diabetes risk: a meta-analysis. Gene 2013;pii: S0378-1119(12)01653-8.
41 Garcia EA, King P, Sidhu K, Ohgusu H, Walley A, Lecoeur C, Gueorguiev M, Khalaf S, Davies D, Grossman AB, Kojima M, Petersenn S, Froguel P, Korbonits M: The role of ghrelin and ghrelin-receptor gene variants and promoter activity in type 2 diabetes. Eur J Endocrinol 2009;161:307–315.
42 Poykko S, Ukkola O, Kauma H, Savolainen MJ, Kesaniemi YA: Ghrelin Arg51Gln mutation is a risk factor for Type 2 diabetes and hypertension in a random sample of middle-aged subjects. Diabetologia 2003;46:455–458.
43 Choi HJ, Cho YM, Moon MK, Choi HH, Shin HD, Jang HC, Kim SY, Lee HK, Park KS: Polymorphisms in the ghrelin gene are associated with serum high-density lipoprotein cholesterol level and not with type 2 diabetes mellitus in Koreans. J Clin Endocrinol Metab 2006;91:4657–4663.

44 Dos Santos ICR, Frigeri HR, Daga DR: The ghrelin gene allele 51Q (rs34911341) is a protective factor against the development of gestational diabetes. Clin Chim Acta 2010;411:886–887.
45 Vartiainen J, Poykko SM, Raisanen T, Kesaniemi YA, Ukkola O: Sequencing analysis of the ghrelin receptor (growth hormone secretagogue receptor type 1a) gene. Eur J Endocrinol 2004;150:457–463.
46 Mager U, Degenhardt T, Pulkkinen L, Kolehmainen M, Tolppanen AM, Lindstrom J, Eriksson JG, Carlberg C, Tuomilehto J, Uusitupa M, Finnish Diabetes Prevention Study Group: Variations in the ghrelin receptor gene associate with obesity and glucose metabolism in individuals with impaired glucose tolerance. PLoSOne 2008;3:e2941.
47 Zou CC, Huang K, Liang L, Zhao ZY: Polymorphisms of the ghrelin/obestatin gene and ghrelin levels in Chinese children with short stature. Clin Endocrinol (Oxf) 2008;69:99–104.
48 Gueorguiev M, Lecoeur C, Benzinou M, Mein CA, Meyre D, Vatin V, Weill J, Heude B, Grossman AB, Froguel P, Korbonits M: A genetic study of the ghrelin and growth hormone secretagogue receptor (GHSR) genes and stature. Ann Hum Genet 2009;73: 1–9.
49 Gueorguiev M, Wiltshire S, Garcia EA, Mein C, Lecoeur C, Kristen B, Allotey R, Hattersley AT, Walker M, O'rahilly S, Froguel P, Grossman AB, McCarthy MI, Hitman GA, Korbonits M: Examining the candidacy of ghrelin as a gene responsible for variation in adult stature in a United Kingdom population with type 2 diabetes. J Clin Endocrinol Metab 2007;92:2201–2204.
50 Garcia EA, Heude B, Petry CJ, Gueorguiev M, Hassan-Smith ZK, Spanou A, Ring SM, Dunger DB, Wareham N, Sandhu MS, Ong KK, Korbonits M: Ghrelin receptor gene polymorphisms and body size in children and adults. J Clin Endocrinol Metab 2008;93:4158–4161.
51 Lango Allen H, Estrada K, Lettre G, et al: Hundreds of variants clustered in genomic loci and biological pathways affect human height. Nature 2010;467: 832–838.
52 Pantel J, Legendre M, Cabrol S, Hilal L, Hajaji Y, Morisset S, Nivot S, Vie-Luton MP, Grouselle D, de Kerdanet M, Kadiri A, Epelbaum J, Le Bouc Y, Amselem S: Loss of constitutive activity of the growth hormone secretagogue receptor in familial short stature. J Clin Invest 2006;116:760–768.
53 Samani NJ, Erdmann J, Hall AS, Hengstenberg C, Mangino M, Mayer B, Dixon RJ, Meitinger T, Braund P, Wichmann HE, Barrett JH, König IR, Stevens SE, Szymczak S, Tregouet DA, Iles MM, Pahlke F, Pollard H, Lieb W, Cambien F, Fischer M, Ouwehand W, Blankenberg S, Balmforth AJ, Baessler A, Ball SG, Strom TM, Braenne I, Gieger C, Deloukas P, Tobin MD, Ziegler A, Thompson JR, Schunkert H, WTCCC and the Cardiogenics Consortium: Genomewide association analysis of coronary artery disease. N Engl J Med 2007;357:443–453.
54 Pantel J, Legendre M, Nivot S, Morisset S, Vie-Luton MP, Le Bouc Y, Epelbaum J, Amselem S: Recessive isolated growth hormone deficiency and mutations in the ghrelin receptor. J Clin Endocrinol Metab 2009;94:4334–4341.
55 Inoue H, Kangawa N, Kinouchi A, Sakamoto Y, Kimura C, Horikawa R, Shigematsu Y, Itakura M, Ogata T, Fujieda K, Japan Growth Genome Consortium: Identification and functional analysis of novel human growth hormone secretagogue receptor (GHSR) gene mutations in Japanese subjects with short stature. J Clin Endocrinol Metab 2011; 96:E373–E378.
56 Pugliese-Pires PN, Fortin JP, Arthur T, Latronico AC, Mendonca BB, Villares SM, Arnhold IJ, Kopin AS, Jorge AA: Novel inactivating mutations in the GH secretagogue receptor gene in patients with constitutional delay of growth and puberty. Eur J Endocrinol 2011;165:233–241.

Professor Márta Korbonits
Centre for Endocrinology, William Harvey Research Institute, John Vane Science Centre
Barts and the London School of Medicine, Queen Mary University of London
Charterhouse square, London EC1M 6BQ (UK)
E-Mail m.korbonits@qmul.ac.uk

Benso A, Casanueva FF, Ghigo E, Granata A (eds): The Ghrelin System.
Endocr Dev. Basel, Karger, 2013, vol 25, pp 41–48 (DOI: 10.1159/000346051)

Ghrelin and the Gut

T.L. Peeters
Gut Peptide Laboratory, Faculty of Medicine, University of Leuven, Leuven, Belgium

Abstract
Ghrelin is the endogenous ligand for the growth hormone secretagogue receptor (GHS-R) which was identified in the pituitary gland and is now named the ghrelin receptor. However, the peptide is most abundant in the stomach and ghrelin receptors are present in all major organ systems and tissues. Ghrelin forms with motilin, a new gut peptide family and the sequence similarities of peptides and receptors suggest they evolved by gene duplication. Nevertheless, no cross-reactivity exits between both peptides. Ghrelin shares with motilin motor effects in the gut, in particular gastric emptying and the induction of the migrating motor complex, but ghrelin also affects gastric acid secretion, offers gastroprotection and may modulate intestinal inflammation. The effects of ghrelin result from the activation of central, vagal and enteric neural receptors and receptors on immune cells. Ghrelin agonists have been developed for the treatment of hypomotility disorders and the peptidomimetic TZP-102 is in phase 2 clinical trials for diabetic gastroparesis.

Relationship of Ghrelin with Motilin

In the context of ghrelin's effects on the gut, the relationship of ghrelin with motilin deserves special attention. When Kojima et al. [1] identified in 1999 ghrelin as the endogenous ligand of the growth hormone secretagogue receptor (GHS-R), they thought ghrelin had no sequence similarity with any known peptide. However, in 2000 another group described the discovery of a peptide with the same sequence which they gave the name motilin-related peptide (MTRLP). Moreover already in 1998 part of the ghrelin sequence was submitted under the name 'motilin homolog' as part of a patent application (for a complete overview of the remarkable history of ghrelin's discovery, see Peeters [2]). Because the sequences of MTRLP and motilin homolog were derived from cDNA sequences, they did not include the octanoylation of serine 3, a distinct feature of ghrelin.[1] Therefore, the true discovery of ghrelin was

[1] Desacylated ghrelin is also secreted and may have biological activities different of those of ghrelin. In the more recent literature, ghrelin is therefore sometimes denoted as 'acylated ghrelin' a pleonasm that should be avoided.

indeed made by Kojima et al. [1], and soon after that discovery it was realized that, considering the sequence similarities, also of their precursors, and of the similar arrangement of their precursors and of their genes, a new peptide family had been discovered as well.

It was also found that the receptors of both peptides are related as well. The ghrelin receptor was originally known as GHS-R. This receptor was discovered in the pituitary gland, due to its activation by growth hormone secretagogues (GHSs), synthetic enkephalin analogues. Shortly before the discovery of ghrelin, the orphan receptor GPR38, structurally related to the GHS-R receptor, was identified as the motilin receptor. The ghrelin, motilin, GPR39, neuromedin U and neurotensin receptors are all structurally related, but the strongest similarity is between the motilin and ghrelin receptors [3].

A detailed analysis of the similarities between motilin and ghrelin, and between their receptors, shows that they evolved by gene duplication but at different points in time [3]. Sharing but also divergence of functions, as exemplified by the species differences in the effects of both peptides, the loss of motilin in rodents, and the opposite motility effect of ghrelin in dog versus man, suggest different functional constraints acting during evolution. This has more than academic importance, as it questions the translational value of animal models in drug development [4].

A 2001 review used as its title 'Ghrelin and motilin: two sides of one coin?' From what is now known about the effects of both peptides, it would perhaps be better to write 'two sides of a loaded coin'. Indeed ghrelin is a pleiotropic peptide affecting almost every system in the body, motilin's effect is not only limited to the gastrointestinal system, but also to motor effects in that system. Ghrelin shares these motor effects but has even on the gut a wider spectrum of effects.

Distribution of Ghrelin Along the Gastrointestinal Tract

Ghrelin is present along the whole gastrointestinal tract with decreasing concentrations from stomach to colon. The distribution of ghrelin mRNA and the distribution the mRNA of ghrelin *O*-acyltransferase (GOAT), the enzyme responsible for the acylation of serine 3, corresponds with the distribution of the peptide. Ghrelin is present in endocrine cells, formerly described in the oxyntic mucosa of the stomach as X/A cells (X for unknown function, A for similarity with pancreatic A cells). They are now named ghrelin cells. They are much more abundant in the gastric body than elsewhere in the gut, and can be open to the lumen, or closed. The open type is more prominent in the lower intestinal tract [5].

From the decreases in plasma levels observed after gastrectomy and small bowel resection it has been estimated that approximately two-thirds of the ghrelin circulating in the plasma is derived from the stomach and the remaining one-third from the small intestine [6].

Receptor Distribution and Cross-Reactivity with Motilin

The ghrelin receptor is present in almost every system and tissue of the body. Localizations playing a role in the effects of ghrelin on the gut will be discussed when considering the mechanism of action. Suffice it to note here that ghrelin receptors are present in several brain regions, in the enteric nervous system, on vagal afferents and in the nodose ganglion.

The activation of the ghrelin receptor involves the transmembrane domains 2 and 3, both well conserved during more than 400 million years of evolution. In particular, glutamic acid residue 124 is critical for binding with ghrelin agonists [7]. The corresponding residue in the motilin receptor plays a similar role suggesting the possibility of cross-reactivity [8].

With regard to the peptides, the biological activity resides in the N-terminal part, an uncommon feature. Apparently, in agreement with this, the amino acid sequences of the N-terminal part are well conserved: in seven mammalian species (human, monkey, cat, dog, pig, sheep, and cow) the first 10 residues in ghrelin are identical, in motilin the first six. Paradoxically, N-terminal fragments retaining appreciable binding affinity must be longer for motilin (about 12) than for ghrelin (only 4). In addition, in ghrelin the most crucial determinant for binding is the octanoylation of serine 3. Thus, sequence similarities do not suggest possible cross-reactivity and as yet no noticeable interactions between ghrelin and motilin agonists have been observed, except a weak affinity of the motilide EM-574 for the ghrelin receptor [4].

Effects of Ghrelin on Gut Function

Gastric Acid Secretion

In the oxyntic mucosa, ghrelin cells are in close proximity to parietal cells and gastrin G cells. A paracrine effect on gastric secretion could be taken into consideration, but has as yet not been demonstrated. Endocrine effects seem to involve vagal and central pathways. Thus, intravenous administration of ghrelin stimulates gastric acid secretion, an effect that is abolished by vagotomy and involves the release of histamine. On the other hand the inhibitory effect of intracerebroventricular ghrelin administration is abolished by cysteamine, suggesting the involvement of a central somatostinergic pathway [2, 9].

Gastroprotection

Ghrelin has a protective effect in models of ethanol- and stress-induced ulcers. The protective effect has been observed as well after intraperitoneal, subcutaneous, or intracerebroventricular administration, suggesting mediation via peripheral and central ghrelin receptors [10]. The protective effects may be due to the production of nitric oxide, prostaglandins, inhibition of the synthesis of pro-inflammatory cytokines or stimulation of the synthesis of anti-inflammatory cytokines. Thus, ghrelin acts directly on enteric neurons to produce nitric oxide (NO) and blockade of NO synthesis blocks this effect. Similarly, blockade of prostaglandin synthesis by indomethacin or the selective COX-2 inhibitor rofecoxib inhibits ghrelin's protective effect (data reviewed in Konturek et al. [10]). Immune B and T cells, monocytes and natural killer cells express ghrelin receptors and ghrelin may be an immunomodulator by affecting the production of cytokines. Indeed ghrelin stimulates the production of the anti-inflammatory cytokines IL-4 and IL-10 and reduces the secretion of pro-inflammatory cytokines such as IL-1α, IL-1β, IL-6 and TNF-α (data reviewed in Stengel and Taché [5]).

The effect of exogenous ghrelin is blocked by a ghrelin antagonist, but the role of endogenous ghrelin has not been investigated, although it has been noted that mucosal expression of ghrelin and ghrelin plasma concentration are increased in stress- and ethanol-induced ulcers [10].

Intestinal Inflammation

From the gastroprotective effects mentioned above and the mechanisms that may be involved, one may assume that ghrelin could have a beneficial effect in inflammatory bowel diseases. Moreover, the increased plasma ghrelin concentration in patients with inflammatory bowel disease and with celiac disease and the rapid rise of plasma ghrelin in response to endotoxin injection in healthy humans [11] may be interpreted as endogenous reactions aimed at countering the inflammatory process. Accordingly, a beneficial effect of a bolus injection of ghrelin was reported in a mouse and rat model of 2,4,6-trinitrobenzenesulfonic acid (TNBS) colitis [12, 13]. However, another study found an adverse effect after prolonged administration of ghrelin. Moreover, in the same study [14] ghrelin KO mice were less susceptible to dextran sulphate sodium (DSS) induced colitis than normal mice. It was suggested that the treatment schedule is at the basis of the different outcomes [14] or the use of DSS versus TNBS [15].

Gastrointestinal Motility

Soon after the discovery of ghrelin, when the relation with motilin became clear, a stimulatory effect on antral motility in rats was described (for an exhaustive review of all motility-related studies with ghrelin, see Sallam and Chen [16]). This observation was also of importance because motilin was known to have no effect in rodents, and this study suggested that the most typical effect of motilin, the induction of the 'migrating motor complex' (MMC), as yet studied mostly in man and dog, could now be studied in small laboratory animals. A detailed study using various routes of administration of ghrelin and ghrelin antagonists showed that in the rat motor effects depend on the activation of central receptors, efferent and afferent vagal pathways [17, 18]. Ghrelin may also have a local effect because ghrelin receptors have been detected in the myenteric plexus of guinea pig ileum and in human and rat stomach and colon. Surprisingly though, ghrelin does not induce an MMC in the dog [19]. Ghrelin even has an inhibitory effect in the dog via an inhibition of the release of motilin. Thus, in physiological conditions the MMC cycle in dog may be coregulated by motilin and ghrelin [20]. This does not appear to be the case in man, where ghrelin was reported to induce an MMC of gastric origin, a typical feature of motilin-induced MMCs, but the effect of ghrelin was not due to a release of motilin [21].

In view of a possible therapeutic application as gastrokinetic the effect of ghrelin on gastric emptying has been received much attention. Ghrelin accelerates gastric emptying in rats, mice and normal human volunteers. Ghrelin also improves delayed gastric emptying in animal models of post-operative ileus, septic ileus, and burn-induced gastroparesis, and in patients with neurogenic, idiopathic or diabetic gastroparesis (data reviewed in De Smet [21]). However, these effects are probably pharmacological. Indeed, ghrelin KO mice have normal gastric emptying [21] and in man low doses of ghrelin, sufficient to stimulate growth hormone release, have no effect on gastric emptying [22]. As for the mechanism of ghrelin-induced acceleration of gastric emptying, one has to rely on mostly indirect studies. Ghrelin activates the enteric nervous system, but in vitro induced contractility is rather weak. In vivo models suggest an important role for vago-vagal reflexes because motor effects are abolished by vagotomy or capsaicin. It should be noted that in mice central administration of ghrelin also accelerates gastric emptying (reviewed in de Smet et al. [21]).

Besides stimulating gastric contractility, gastrokinetics may also inhibit gastric accommodation by increasing fundic tone and in this way induce adverse symptoms and early satiety. This may have been one of the reasons why motilin agonists worsened symptoms in patients with gastroparesis and therefore failed in clinical trials. It is of interest to note that ghrelin also inhibits gastric accommodation, but does not induce adverse effects or satiety. This may be due to the fact that ghrelin combines peripheral effects such as increased antral contractility and fundic tone, with central effects modulating vagally mediated symptom sensation and that the known centrally mediated orexigenic effect may override the satiety signal generated by the increased fundic tone [23].

Pathophysiology

Under normal conditions ghrelin plasma levels increase before and decrease after a meal [6], making comparisons between patient groups difficult. The mechanisms controlling these fluctuations are also poorly understood making interpretations of observed differences, on a larger time scale, difficult. For example, plasma ghrelin is increased in anorexic and cachectic patients and decreased in obese patients [5], the opposite of what one would expect, but perhaps the result of a mechanism counteracting the appetite stimulating effect of ghrelin.

Reports on changes in plasma ghrelin in gastrointestinal diseases have been compiled by El-Salhy [11]. Increased levels were reported in IBD, functional dyspepsia, celiac disease, after vagotomy and after *Helicobacter* eradication, decreased levels in gastritis, gastric ulcer, gastrectomy, small bowel resection, and gastric bypass surgery. However, a causal relationship between plasma ghrelin changes and the pathological condition is lacking, except that it seems logical that removal of the ghrelin-producing mucosa, as in gastrectomy, or damage to the mucosa, as in *Helicobacter pylori* infection may lead to a reduction of ghrelin production. In *H. pylori* infection this may contribute to the development of ulcers. After eradication, one study noted a rise of plasma ghrelin, but this was not confirmed in another study based on a larger group of patients. The discrepancy may be explained by the different topography (antrum or fundus, where ghrelin cells are located) and duration of the infection (reversible damage after a short infection, irreversible atrophy after long infection) in both studies [2]. The issue may be important because it has been suggested that eradication of *H. pylori*, via its effect on plasma ghrelin, may contribute to the development of obesity and may also increase the risk of esophageal adenocarcinoma [24].

As described above, ghrelin inhibits gastric accommodation suggesting a possible role of ghrelin. Therefore, plasma levels of ghrelin have been studied in patients in comparison with controls and in relation to gastric emptying, symptom score and psychological factors. The results, recently summarized by Ogiso et al. [25], are conflicting and contradictory. It seems safe to conclude that ghrelin does not play a major role in the pathophysiology of functional dyspepsia.

Ghrelin Agonists for Motility Disorders

Growth hormone secretagogues, now known to be ghrelin agonists, were developed for the treatment of growth hormone deficiency but failed in clinical trials. Some of them, such as GHRP-6 and ipamorelin, are now being reevaluated as prokinectics. Ipamorelin is in phase 2b development for postoperative ileus (Helsinn Pharmaceuticals). The same company lists a further unspecified compound, ST-1141, in phase 1 development for opioid induced bowel dysfunction (http://www.helsinn.com).

Macrocyclic peptidomimetics with ghrelin agonist activity and chemically distinct from the GHS were developed by Tranzyme. TZP-101, now named ulimorelin, is a compound for intravenous use. It does stimulate gastric emptying but not growth hormone release. It was developed for postoperative ileus and showed promising results in phase 2 studies but failed to meet primary and secondary endpoints in the first of two phase 3 trials. In March 2012, the company announced that development of

TZP-101 was stopped. The company next concentrate on TZP-102, an orally active compound granted fast track status by the FDA. However end December 2012 development of TZP-102 was stopped because of a lack of efficacy. Apparently ghrelin also shares with motilin the difficulty to let the prokinetic properties of its agonists become a benefit to patients.

References

1 Kojima M, Hosoda H, Date Y, Nakazato M, Matsuo H, Kangawa K: Ghrelin is a growth-hormone-releasing acylated peptide from stomach. Nature 1999;402: 656–660.

2 Peeters TL: Ghrelin: a new player in the regulation of gastrointestinal function. Gut 2005;54:1638–1649.

3 He J, Irwin DM, Zhang Y-P: The power of an evolutionary perspective in studies of endocrinology; in Diamanti-Kandarakis E (ed): Contemporary Aspects of Endocrinology. 2011. InTech, Available from: http://www.intechopen.com/books/contemporary-aspects-ofendocrinology/the-power-of-an-evolutionary-perspective-in-studies-of-endocrinology.

4 Sanger GJ, Holbrook JD, Andrews PLR: The translational value of rodent gastrointestinal functions: a cautionary tale. Trends Pharmacol Sci 2011;32:402–409.

5 Stengel A, Taché Y: Ghrelin – a pleiotropic hormone secreted from endocrineX/A-like cells of the stomach. Front Neurosci 2012:6:1–16.

6 Cummings DE: *Helicobacter pylori* and ghrelin: interrelated players in body-weight regulation? Am J Med 2004;117:436–439.

7 Feighner SD, Howard AD, Prendergast K, Palyha OC, Hreniuk DL, Nargund R, Underwood D, Tata JR, Dean DC, Tan CP, McKee KK, Woods JW, Patchett AA, Smith RG, Van der Ploeg LH: Structural requirements for the activation of the human growth hormone secretagogue receptor by peptide and nonpeptide secretagogues. Mol Endocrinol 1998;12:137–145.

8 Xu L, Depoortere I, Vertongen P, Waelbroeck M, Robberecht P, Peeters TL: Motilin and erythromycin: a share a common binding site in the third transmembrane segment of the motilin receptor. Biochem Pharmacol 2005;70:879–887.

9 Yakabi K, Kawashima J, Kato S: Ghrelin and gastric acid secretion. World J Gastroenterol 2008;14:6334–6338.

10 Konturek PC, Brzozowski T, Pajdo R, Nikiforuk A, Kwiecien S, Harsch I, Drozdowicz D, Hahn EG, Konturek SJ: Ghrelin – a new gastroprotective factor in gastric mucosa. J Physiol Pharmacol 2004;55:325–336.

11 El-Salhy M: Ghrelin in gastrointestinal diseases and disorders: a possible role in the pathophysiology and clinical implications (review). Int J Mol Med 2009; 24:727–732.

12 Gonzalez-Rey E, Chorny A, Delgado M: Therapeutic action of ghrelin in a mouse model of colitis. Gastroenterology 2006;130:1707–1720.

13 Konturek PC, Brzozowski T, Engel M: Ghrelin ameliorates colonic inflammation. Role of nitric oxide and sensory nerves. J Physiol Pharmacol 2009;60: 41–47.

14 De Smet B, Thijs T, Moechars D, Colsoul B, Polders L, Ver Donck L, Coulie B, Peeters TL, Depoortere I: Endogenous and exogenous ghrelin enhance the colonic and gastric manifestations of dextran sodium sulphate-induced colitis in mice. Neurogastrenterol Motil 2009;21:59–70.

15 Deboer MD: Use of ghrelin as a treatment for inflammatory bowel disease: mechanistic considerations. Int J Pept 2011;2011:189242.

16 Sallam HS, Chen JZ: The prokinetic face of ghrelin. Int J Peptides 2010;2010 pii:493614.

17 Fujino K, Inui A, Asakawa A, Kihara N, Fujimura M, Fujimiya M: Ghrelin induces fasted motor activity of the gastrointestinal tract in conscious fed rats. J Physiol 2003;550:227–240.

18 Page AJ, Slattery JA, Milte C, Laker R, O'donnell T, Dorian C: Ghrelin selectively reduces mechanosensitivity of upper gastrointestinal vagal afferents. Am J Physiol Gastrointest Liver Physiol 2007;292:G1376–G1384.

19 Ohno T, Kamiyama Y, Aihara R, Nakabayashi T, Mochiki E, Asao T, Kuwano H: Ghrelin does not stimulate gastrointestinal motility and gastric emptying: an experimental study of conscious dogs. Neurogastroenterol Motil 2006;18:129–135.

20 Ogawa A, Mochiki E, Yanai M, Morita H, Toyomasu Y, Ogata K, Ohno T, Asao T, Kuwano H: Interdigestive migrating contractions are coregulated by ghrelin and motilin in conscious dogs. Am J Physiol 2012; 302:R233–R243.

21 De Smet B, Mitselos A, Depoortere I: Motilin and ghrelin as prokinetic drug targets. Pharmacol Ther 2009;123:207–223.

22 Cremonini F, Camilleri M, Vazquez Roque M, Mckinzie S, Burton D, Baxter K: Obesity does not increase effects of synthetic ghrelin on human gastric motor functions. Gastroenterology 2006;131:1431–1439.
23 Ang D, Nicolai H, Vos R, Mimidis K, Akyuz F, Kindt S, Vanden Berghe P, Sifrim D, Depoortere I, Peeters T, Tack J: Influence of ghrelin on the gastric accommodation reflex and on meal-induced satiety in man. Neurogastroenterol Motil 2009;21:528–533.
24 Nwokolo CU, Freshwater DA, O'Hare P, Randeva HS: Plasma ghrelin following cure of Helicobacter pylori. Gut 2003;52:637–640.
25 Ogiso K, Asakawa A, Amitani H, Inui A: Ghrelin: a gut hormonal basis of motility regulation and functional dyspepsia. J Gastroenterol Hepatol 2011;suppl 3:67–72.

T.L. Peeters
Gut Peptide Laboratory, Faculty of Medicine, University of Leuven
Kasteeldreef 38
BE–3210 Lubbeek (Linden) (Belgium)
E-Mail theo.peeters@med.kuleuven.be

Benso A, Casanueva FF, Ghigo E, Granata A (eds): The Ghrelin System.
Endocr Dev. Basel, Karger, 2013, vol 25, pp 49–58 (DOI: 10.1159/000346052)

Ghrelin as a GH-Releasing Factor

M.C. Carreira[a] · A.B. Crujeiras[a] · S. Andrade[b, c] · M.P. Monteiro[b] · F.F. Casanueva[a, b]

[a]CIBER de Fisiopatologia Obesidad y Nutricion (CB06/03), Instituto Salud Carlos III and [b]Department of Medicine, Santiago de Compostela University, Complejo Hospitalario Universitario de Santiago (CHUS), Santiago de Compostela, Spain; [c]Department of Anatomy and UMIB (Unit for Multidisciplinary Biomedical Research) of ICBAS, University of Porto, Porto, Portugal

Abstract

Growth hormone (GH) is secreted by the pituitary gland in a pulsatile manner. It is accepted that this pulsatility is primarily controlled by the hypothalamus, although this secretion can also be modulated by factors from GH-targeted organs, the pituitary and other regions of the central nervous systems, or by factors arriving from peripheral organs. In mammals, hypothalamic control of GH pulsatility is classically regulated by the interplay of two opposing hormones, stimulatory GHRH and inhibitory somatostatin (SS). Recognition of the gastric ghrelin peptide as the natural ligand for GH secretagogue receptor type 1a (GHS-R1a) added a new element to the complex physiological regulation of GH secretion and clarified some of its aspects that were previously not fully understood. In this review, we examine data that suggest that ghrelin may regulate GH secretion, as well as ghrelin's possible use as a therapeutic agent.

The discovery of ghrelin began with the research of Bowers and collaborators, who demonstrated that small synthetic peptides, which are structurally based on met-encephalin, stimulate and amplify pulsatile growth hormone (GH) release; they named these GH-releasing peptides (GHRPs) [1]. Later, synthetic nonpeptidic molecules, such as MK-0677, were also shown to be able to induce GH release, probably through the same nonidentified receptor [2]. The peptidic and nonpeptidic molecules with GH-releaser activities were known by the general term of GH secretagogues (GHS). In the 1990s, the use of MK-0677 allowed for the cloning of the endogenous receptor to which GHS binds, a typical seven-transmembrane G protein-coupled receptor that belongs to the superfamily of motilin, neurotensin and neuromedin receptors, and this receptor was named GH secretagogue receptor 1a (GHS-R1a) [3]. There are two GHS-R molecules identified currently: GHS-R1a and GHS-R1b. The 1a isoform me-

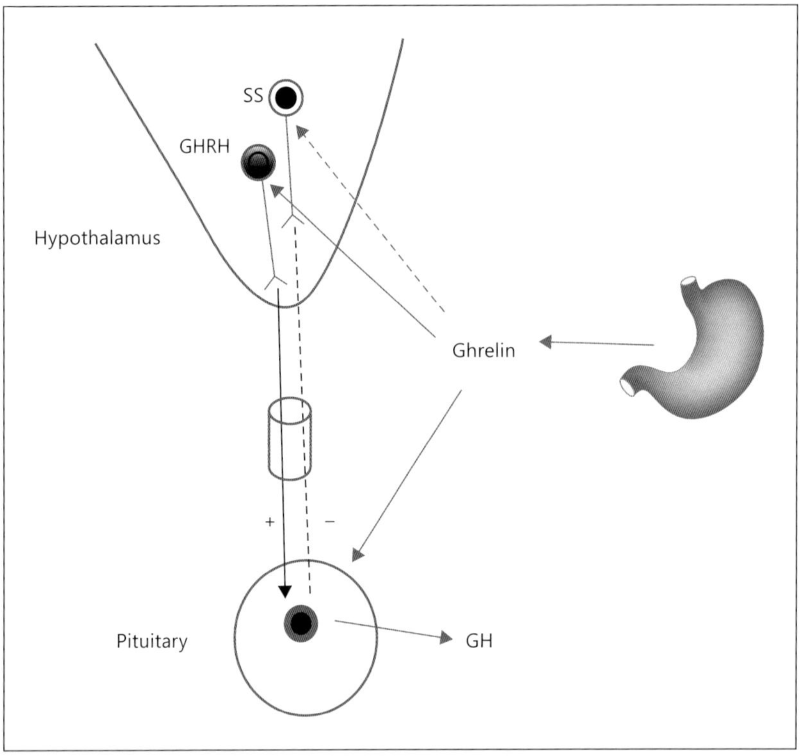

Fig. 1. Schematic representation of ghrelin production and action on the central nervous system to stimulate GH release. Solid line = Stimulatory effect; dotted line = inhibitory effect.

diates GH-releasing orexigenic effects, and is found in the hypothalamus, including the arcuate and ventromedial nuclei, in the pituitary gland and in other tissues, especially those of endocrine origin. In contrast, the 1b isoform is produced by alternative splicing of pre-mRNA from the GHSR gene in a multitude of tissues, but its significance is not clear [6, 11].

Finally, ghrelin, the endogenous ligand for this receptor, was identified in 1999 [4]. Ghrelin is expressed abundantly in specialized cells in the oxyntic gland of the gastric epithelium [5] (fig. 1). In addition, low-level ghrelin expression also occurs in several tissues, including the hypothalamus, pituitary, lung, pancreas, adrenal cortex, thyroid, kidney, testis and placenta [4, 6, 8]. Ghrelin is a 28-amino acid peptide and undergoes posttranslational octanoylation of serine 3 catalyzed by ghrelin *O*-acyltransferase (GOAT) [9, 10], a modification that is essential for the endocrine actions of ghrelin [6]. The peptide is rapidly deacylated by circulating enzymes producing des-acyl ghrelin, which is present in higher concentrations than the acylated form in the tissues and blood. Although it is unable to bind to GHS-R1a and is devoid of endocrine actions, des-acyl ghrelin is biologically active as a regulator in the prostate, in adipogenesis and in the cardiovascular system [6]. Des-acyl ghrelin has also been implicated in the regulation of glucose homeostasis, inhibiting the effects of acyl ghrelin on insulin secretion from rodent pancreas isolated islets [7]. Interestingly, the effects of ghrelin and des-acyl ghrelin on insulin are abolished by co-administration of both peptides [7] suggesting that these actions of des-acyl ghrelin are mediated by a receptor other than GHS-R1a. However, the des-acyl ghrelin has similar effects to acyl ghrelin on lipid metabolism, promoting lipogenesis in vivo and inhibiting lipolysis in rat adipoctyes [7].

GH Secretion and Role of Ghrelin

GH is produced and secreted by the somatotrope cells of the anterior pituitary, although it is accepted that other extrapituitary sites produce GH with autocrine or paracrine actions [6, 11]. GH secretion is pulsatile in all mammal species studied with a sexual dimorphic pattern. This pulsatility is mainly controlled by the hypothalamus, and can also be modulated by several factors produced in the pituitary, in other regions of the central nervous system or in peripheral regions. At the hypothalamic level, GH secretion in mammals is controlled in a dual manner by two peptides with opposing roles, GH-releasing hormone (GHRH) and somatotropin release-inhibiting factor (SRIF, or somatostatin). However, this dual model is too simple, and it is not completely supported by the data [6, 11, 12], suggesting important GH-regulatory roles for additional peptides at the hypothalamic level, and ghrelin might represent an interesting third player in GH regulation (fig. 1).

In accordance with the identification of ghrelin as the endogenous ligand for GH secretagogue receptors, initial studies with exogenous synthetic GH secretagogues and ghrelin have shown a strong and dose-dependent GH-releasing effect [4] that potentially includes activity at the pituitary and/or hypothalamus (fig. 1).

The effect of ghrelin in vivo is stronger than in vitro, and it is dependent on the presence of GHRH. Moreover, ghrelin shows an additive or even synergistic effect on GHRH-stimulated GH release and prevents cyclic refractoriness to GHRH. In addition, ghrelin-mediated GH secretion is reduced, although not completely abolished, in animals with lesions of the pituitary stalk, suggesting that the main action of ghrelin occurs at hypothalamus [11, 13]. In any case, the sources of ghrelin for GH-releasing effects could be multiple. Systemic ghrelin of gastric origin is the first option. It is also plausible that hypothalamic ghrelin could be involved in GH regulation via secretion into the hypophyseal-portal blood or modulation of hypothalamic GHRH and/or SS expression or action. In contrast, pituitary-produced ghrelin could improve somatotrope cells sensitivity to GHRH. In this sense, ghrelin expression in the pituitary suggests an autocrine or paracrine role in GH regulation. In fact, under experimental conditions in which hypothalamic GHRH expression is increased (GH or glucocorticoid deficiency, hypothyroidism), pituitary ghrelin levels are also increased [14]. Consistent with this correlation, pituitary ghrelin expression levels are decreased in con-

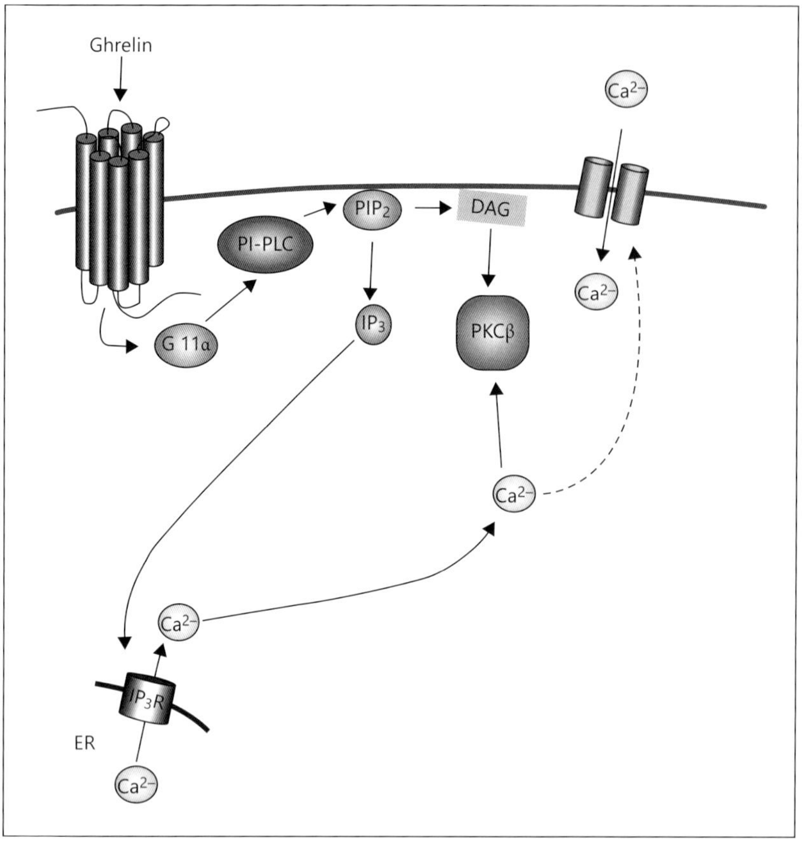

Fig. 2. The signal transduction pathway activated by ghrelin through the GHS-R1a receptor. The binding of ghrelin to the GHS-R 1a activates the subunit G 11α of the G protein and phospholipase C (PLC) signaling pathway, resulting in hydrolysis of membrane-bound phosphatidylinositol biphosphate (PIP_2) to inositol triphosphate (IP_3) and DAG. DAG activates protein kinase C, inhibiting K^+ channels and depolarizing somatotrope cells, which results in the opening of voltage-dependent channels and IP_3-mediated release of calcium from the endoplasmic reticulum (ER), leading to GH secretion.

ditions in which hypothalamic GHRH expression is decreased, indicating a physiological role for GHRH in stimulating pituitary ghrelin levels [14, 15].

Some evidence supports the idea that the presence of GHRH is necessary for ghrelin-mediated GH release. GHS and ghrelin administration induces *c-fos* expression and electrical activity in the arcuate nucleus in vivo and in vitro, and GHRH neurons express GHS-R1a [6, 12, 15]. Pretreatment with GHRH antiserum or GHRH-R antagonists blocks GH response to different GHS in humans and rodents [6, 12, 15]. Humans with GHRH-R mutations or lit/lit mice show low responses to GHS [6, 12, 15].

The signal transduction pathway activated by ghrelin through GHS-R (fig. 2) involves phospholipase C (PLC), resulting in hydrolysis of membrane-bound phosphatidylinositol biphosphate (PIP_2) to inositol triphosphate (IP_3) and diacylglycerol (DAG). DAG activates protein kinase C, inhibiting K^+ channels and depolarizing somatotrope cells, which results in the opening of voltage-dependent channels and IP_3-mediated release of calcium from the endoplasmic reticulum, evoking GH secretion and, perhaps, GHRH release [3, 8, 15]. Although this is the main signaling pathway used by ghrelin, ghrelin is able to modestly increase cAMP levels, which explains GH secretion in response to ghrelin and GHS in models of GHRH deficiency. In contrast, GHRH, through its specific 7-transmembrane G protein coupled receptor, stimulates adenylate cyclase, increasing intracellular cAMP levels, which induce GH synthesis and release. The interaction between ghrelin- and GHRH-signaling pathways and their subsequent effects is not clear. Direct interaction between GHRH-R and GHS-R in pituitary somatotropes has been proposed [16]. Moreover, the recent identification of GHRH as an allosteric modulator of GHS-R1a, as well as of ghrelin binding and potency, provides an explanation for the complementary actions of GHRH and ghrelin and suggests a new mechanism of regulation [17].

Taking into account its strong and reproducible GH-releasing effect, particularly when combined with GHRH, ghrelin can be used as a diagnostic tool in suspected GH deficiency. Ghrelin, when administrated together with GHRH, exerts synergistic action on GH secretion, and this combination is the most potent GH releaser actually known [6, 11, 13]. Clinical studies have demonstrated that ghrelin and GHRH co-administration might be considered a test of GH reserve in humans because the GH response elicited is not altered by sex, age or adiposity. This test is able to discriminate between healthy subjects and patients with GH deficiency. In this condition, the somatotrope response to ghrelin is reduced, while the lactotrope and corticotrope responses are fully preserved [6, 11, 13]. These results suggest that ghrelin might be used as a reliable test to evaluate maximal secretory capacity, although they do not support the idea that impaired ghrelin response is the major cause of GH deficiency.

In addition, it has been proposed that ghrelin rejuvenates the GH/IGF-1 axis, with possible clinical applications in aging because chronic administration of ghrelin can increase age-related low GH levels [6, 11, 13].

Does Circulating Ghrelin Act on GH Secretion Control?

Although it has been demonstrated in several experimental studies that ghrelin administration stimulates GH release in vivo and in vitro through a hypothalamus-pituitary mechanism, it is not clear that circulating ghrelin plays a real role in physiological GH secretion.

Taking into consideration that ghrelin levels increase during the nighttime, it appears obvious that this increase could be an explanation for the nocturnal increase of GH secretion. However, such a correlation between ghrelin and GH maximums is not clear [12]. Immunoneutralization of ghrelin abolishes the GH response to exogenous ghrelin without an alteration in endogenous GH pulsatility, whereas GHRH immunoneutralization completely abolishes GH pulsatility in rats, suggesting that ghrelin does not play a key role in GH release. Administration of GHS antagonists does not alter GH pulsatility but decreases pulse amplitude, suggesting synergism of GHS with GHRH. Other studies have found a reduction in circulating ghrelin during fasting-associated GH increases, as opposed to the expectation that, if circulating, ghrelin was responsible for this increase in GH levels [12]. In humans submitted to gastric bypass surgery with very low ghrelin levels, GH secretion is normal.

Data from genetically altered animal models are also conflicting. Ghrelin null mice (knockout) present a tendency toward low IGF-1 levels but normal growth compared with wild-type animals. In contrast, GHS-R knockout mice have low IGF-1 levels and modestly decreased weight compared with control animals. The modest changes observed in these models could be explained by the presence of a redundant system and/or to the high constitutive activity of the GHS-R1a receptor, which is very active even in situations of lack of ghrelin [18, 19]. In humans, a mis-sense mutation, which impairs the constitutive signaling of the GHSR-1a but preserves ghrelin-mediated signal transduction, is associated with short stature [20].

Overall, the data regarding the role of circulating ghrelin as a key regulator of GH secretion are not clear. In this sense, it is important to note that most of the available studies and techniques measure total ghrelin and do not distinguish between ghrelin and des-acyl ghrelin, the circulating concentration of which far exceeds that of the acylated and GH-releasing active forms (approximately 10% of circulating immunoreactivity). Moreover, the measurement of circulating ghrelin does not include the possibility that hypothalamic- or pituitary-produced ghrelin could be involved in the control of GH secretion.

Interactions between Ghrelin and Obestatin to Regulate GH Secretion

Obestatin is a 23-amino acid amidated peptide derived from the C-terminal portion of the 117-amino acid prepro-ghrelin precursor [21]. It was originally thought that obestatin binds to the G protein-associated receptor GPR 39, and it was postulated as a physiological opponent of ghrelin that inhibited food intake and weight gain [21]. However, the effects of this peptide on food intake currently remain unclear. In addition, obestatin is able to produce several biological functions at the central level, such as improving memory, anxiolysis and activation of cortical neurons, as well as peripheral effects. At the cellular level, obestatin stimulates GH release from rat tumor somatotrope cells.

The co-administration in rodents of ghrelin and obestatin at equimolar quantities inhibits the effects of ghrelin alone [22, 23]. This effect could be mediated by the interaction of obestatin and ghrelin at the hypothalamic level, and this process appears not to be mediated by GPR39 because inhibition is maintained in the absence of

GPR39 in the mouse hypothalamus [21]. However, it is important to clarify the significance of this inhibition and the circulating concentrations of both peptides under physiological conditions. It was previously reported that ghrelin and obestatin presented equimolar concentrations in rat and mouse plasma. In another study, obestatin concentrations were much lower, with a ghrelin-to-obestatin ratio of 400:1 [23, 24]. In contrast, obestatin competes with ghrelin for GHS-R1a in pancreatic β-cell lines, suggesting an interaction of obestatin with GHS-R1a receptor [25].

Ghrelin and GH in Elderly

Aging is associated with a severe decrease in circulating GH levels, which is already observed from the second decade of life and is accompanied by catabolic effects, such as a decrease in lean mass, an increase in fat mass and a decrease in bone density, among others. These symptoms are manifestations of complex changes involving the GH axis, for which aging could be defined as somatopause. For this reason, it is possible to suggest that an anabolic drug with GH-releasing effects might play a therapeutic role for antiaging purposes in elderly subjects. If this drug were an orally active compound, the increase in GHS caused by its application would make it a potentially therapeutic molecule. The GH-releasing effects of GHS are age-dependent, increasing during puberty and decreasing with aging. In accordance with the reduction of GHS-R expression at the hypothalamic level in human aging, the GH response to GHS is reduced. This effect could be mediated by GHRH hypoactivity and/or somatostatin hyperactivity. In addition, it is also suggested that age-related reductions in GH levels might be due to a decrease in the ghrelin/GHSR system [6, 11–13]. In fact, acyl-ghrelin levels are lower in elderly adults, compared to young adults. Interestingly, the pituitary level of GHSR does not decline with aging, and the GH release of the pituitary in response to ghrelin and GHS is not altered. Ghrelin and GHS administration increase GH pulses and IGF-1 concentrations, reaching levels equivalent to those in young adults. In addition, several studies have also suggested a role for ghrelin in the treatment of anorexia and sarcopenia during aging. The administration of synthetic GHS increases lean body mass but does not change muscle strength or function [6, 11–13].

Pharmacology of the Ghrelin/GHS-R1a System

The GH-releasing properties of ghrelin are interesting for the treatment of physiological (aging) and pathological (cancer, GH deficiency, cachexia) causes associated with low GH levels. However, it is necessary to take into consideration that ghrelin is a highly pleiotropic hormone with a lipolytic effect via GH release and a fat storage promoter effect via increases in food intake and adipogenesis and decreases in lipid utilization. This means that its effects must be tested to prevent undesirable effects.

Because of its pleiotropic activity, ghrelin or its analogs, especially orally active compounds such as MK-0677, could be a plausible option for several therapies. The administration of MK-0677 to aging subjects recovers the amplitude of GH pulses to similar levels to those of young adults, with increasing lean mass and bone density. The recent ghrelin analog TZP-101, with a high affinity for the GHS-R1a receptor, stimulates food intake but not GH secretion after a central peripheral injection in rodents [26]. This effect appears to be due to the ability of the GHS-R1a receptor to respond in a different manner and the function of the concentration or its agonist molecular/tridimensional structure. These data raise the possibility of developing drugs with specific effects that can differentiate between ghrelin-mediated actions.

In contrast, GHS-R1a antagonists can distinguish the roles of ghrelin under physiological and pathological situations and the effects of ghrelin on GH secretion and food intake. The specific GHS-R1a antagonist BIM-28163 reduces GH secretory pulses but not food intake [27]. In addition, BIM-28163 also exerts agonistic activities, stimulating food intake and weight gain. Another antagonist, JMV2810, can antagonize the effects of hexarelin on food intake but not alter the GH secretion [28]. Considering that ghrelin-mediated GH secretion and ghrelin's orexigenic actions are mediated by the GHS-R1a receptor, these data reveal that GHS-R1a could lead to diverse effects from different levels of activation. At the molecular level, these differences could include constitutive activities, different signaling pathways or allosteric/ago-allosteric mechanisms. In any case, this phenomenon is very interesting, allowing for the future development of the pharmacological dissociation of ghrelin's effects, depending on the desired effects.

Concluding Remarks

Ghrelin is secreted from the stomach into the circulation but is also synthesized in a large number of endocrine and nonendocrine tissues, suggesting a possible dual role for ghrelin as an autocrine and/or endocrine factor. The complete role of circulating ghrelin levels in GH secretion is still controversial. Several data suggest that ghrelin plays a role in the regulation of the GH secretion pattern, in addition to GHRH and somatostatin, particularly by increasing GH peaks before food intake. In contrast, although ghrelin and obestatin interact to modulate GH secretion, it is necessary to characterize their specific contributions. In addition, there is a pressing need to develop more sensitive and selective assays to detect active ghrelin and the different preproghrelin peptides. A better understanding of the regulation of ghrelin gene transcription and of these genes' ratios and their roles, including under varying physiological and pathological conditions, could be the key to developing future therapies.

References

1 Bowers CY, Chang J, Momany FA, Folkers K: Effect of enkephalins and enkephalins analogs on release of pituitary hormones in vitro. Mol Endocrinol 1977: 287–292.

2 Bowers CY: Unnatural growth hormone-releasing peptide begets natural ghrelin. J Clin Endocrinol Metab 2001;86:1464–1469.

3 Howard AD, Feighner SD, Cully DF, Arena JP, Liberator PA, Rosenblum CI, Hamelin M, Hreniuk DL, Palyha OC, Anderson J, Paress PS, Diaz C, Chou M, Liu KK, McKee KK, Pong SS, Chaung LY, Elbrecht A, Dashkevicz M, Heavens R, Rigby M, Sirinathsinghji DJ, Dean DC, Melillo DG, Patchett AA, Nargund R, Griffin PR, DeMartino JA, Gupta SK, Schaeffer JM, Smith RG, Van der Ploeg LH: A receptor in pituitary and hypothalamus that functions in growth hormone release. Science 1996;273:974–977.

4 Kojima M, Hosoda H, Date Y, Nakazato M, Matsuo H, Kangawa K: Ghrelin is a growth-hormone-releasing acylated peptide from stomach. Nature 1999;402: 656–660.

5 Date Y, Kojima M, Hosoda H, Sawaguchi A, Mondal MS, Suganuma T, Matsukura S, Kangawa K, Nakazato M: Ghrelin, a novel growth hormone-releasing acylated peptide, is synthesized in a distinct endocrine cell type in the gastrointestinal tracts of rats and humans. Endocrinology 2000;141:4255–4261.

6 van der Lely AJ, Tschöp M, Heiman ML, Ghigo E: Biological, physiological, pathophysiological, and pharmacological aspects of ghrelin. Endocr Rev 2004;25:426–457.

7 Soares JB, Leite-Moreira AF: Ghrelin, des-acyl ghrelin and obestatin: three pieces of the same puzzle. Peptides 2008;29:1255–1270.

8 Fukushima N, Hanada R, Teranishi H, Fukue Y, Tachibana T, Ishikawa H, Takeda S, Takeuchi Y, Fukumoto S, Kangawa K, Nagata K, Kojima M: Ghrelin directly regulates bone formation. J Bone Miner Res 2005;20:790–798.

9 Gutierrez JA, Solenberg PJ, Perkins DR, Willency JA, Knierman MD, Jin Z, Witcher DR, Luo S, Onyia JE, Hale JE: Ghrelin octanoylation mediated by an orphan lipid transferase. Proc Natl Acad Sci USA 2008; 105:6320–6325.

10 Yang J, Brown MS, Liang G, Grishin NV, Goldstein JL: Identification of the acyltransferase that octanoylates ghrelin, an appetite-stimulating peptide hormone. Cell 2008;132:387–396.

11 Korbonits M, Goldstone AP, Gueorguiev M, Grossman AB: Ghrelin – a hormone with multiple functions. Front Neuroendocrinol 2004;25:27–68.

12 Nass R, Gaylinn BD, Thorner MO: The role of ghrelin in GH secretion and GH disorders. Mol Cell Endocrinol 2011;340:10–14.

13 Casanueva FF, Dieguez C: Ghrelin: the link connecting growth with metabolism and energy homeostasis. Rev Endocr Metab Disord 2002;3:325–338.

14 Kamegai J, Tamura H, Shimizu T, Ishii S, Tatsuguchi A, Sugihara H, Oikawa S, Kineman RD: The role of pituitary ghrelin in growth hormone (GH) secretion: GH-releasing hormone-dependent regulation of pituitary ghrelin gene expression and peptide content. Endocrinology 2004;145:3731–3738.

15 Bennett PA, Thomas GB, Howard AD, Feighner SD, van der Ploeg LH, Smith RG, Robinson IC: Hypothalamic growth hormone secretagogue-receptor (GHS-R) expression is regulated by growth hormone in the rat. Endocrinology 1997;138:4552–4557.

16 Cunha SR, Mayo KE: Ghrelin and growth hormone (GH) secretagogues potentiate GH-releasing hormone (GHRH)-induced cyclic adenosine 3″,5″-monophosphate production in cells expressing transfected GHRH and GH secretagogue receptors. Endocrinology 2002;143:4570–4582.

17 Casanueva FF, Camiña JP, Carreira MC, Pazos Y, Varga JL, Schally AV: Growth hormone-releasing hormone as an agonist of the ghrelin receptor GHS-R1a. Proc Natl Acad Sci USA 2008;105:20452–20457.

18 Sun Y, Ahmed S, Smith RG: Deletion of ghrelin impairs neither growth nor appetite. Mol Cell Biol 2003; 23:7973–7981.

19 Sun Y, Wang P, Zheng H, Smith RG: Ghrelin stimulation of growth hormone release and appetite is mediated through the growth hormone secretagogue receptor. Proc Natl Acad Sci USA 2004;101:4679–4684.

20 Pantel J, Legendre M, Cabrol S, Hilal L, Hajaji Y, Morisset S, Nivot S, Vie-Luton MP, Grouselle D, de Kerdanet M, Kadiri A, Epelbaum J, Le Bouc Y, Amselem S: Loss of constitutive activity of the growth hormone secretagogue receptor in familial short stature. J Clin Invest 2006;116:760–768.

21 Zhang JV, Ren PG, Avsian-Kretchmer O, Luo CW, Rauch R, Klein C, Hsueh AJ: Obestatin, a peptide encoded by the ghrelin gene, opposes ghrelin's effects on food intake. Science 2005;310:996–999.

22 Nogueiras R, Pfluger P, Tovar S, Arnold M, Mitchell S, Morris A, Perez-Tilve D, Vázquez MJ, Wiedmer P, Castañeda TR, DiMarchi R, Tschöp M, Schurmann A, Joost HG, Williams LM, Langhans W, Diéguez C: Effects of obestatin on energy balance and growth hormone secretion in rodents. Endocrinology 2007; 148:21–26.

23 Zizzari P, Longchamps R, Epelbaum J, Bluet-Pajot MT: Obestatin partially affects ghrelin stimulation of food intake and growth hormone secretion in rodents. Endocrinology 2007;148:1648–1653.

24 Hassouna R, Zizzari P, Tolle V: The ghrelin/obestatin balance in the physiological and pathological control of growth hormone secretion, body composition and food intake. J Neuroendocrinol 2010;22:793–804.
25 Granata R, Settanni F, Gallo D, Trovato L, Biancone L, Cantaluppi V, Nano R, Annunziata M, Campiglia P, Arnoletti E, Ghè C, Volante M, Papotti M, Muccioli G, Ghigo E: Obestatin promotes survival of pancreatic beta-cells and human islets and induces expression of genes involved in the regulation of beta-cell mass and function. Diabetes 2008;57:967–979.
26 Fraser GL, Hoveyda HR, Tannenbaum GS, Fraser GL, Hoveyda HR: Pharmacological demarcation of the growth hormone, gut motility and feeding effects of ghrelin using a novel ghrelin receptor agonist. Endocrinology 2008;149:6280–6288.
27 Halem HA, Taylor JE, Dong JZ, Shen Y, Datta R, Abizaid A, Diano S, Horvath TL, Culler MD: A novel growth hormone secretagogue-1a receptor antagonist that blocks ghrelin-induced growth hormone secretion but induces increased body weight gain. Neuroendocrinology 2005;81:339–349.
28 Demange L, Boeglin D, Moulin A, Mousseaux D, Ryan J, Bergé G, Gagne D, Heitz A, Perrissoud D, Locatelli V, Torsello A, Galleyrand JC, Fehrentz JA, Martinez J: Synthesis and pharmacological in vitro and in vivo evaluations of novel triazole derivatives as ligands of the ghrelin receptor. J Med Chem 2007;50:1939–1957.

F.F. Casanueva
Laboratorio de Endocrinología Molecular nº 2, Instituto de Investigaciones Sanitarias de Santiago de Compostela
Planta -2, Complexo Hospitalario Universitario de Santiago, Travesía da Choupana s/n
ES–15706 Santiago de Compostela (Spain)
E-Mail felipe.casanueva@usc.es

Benso A, Casanueva FF, Ghigo E, Granata A (eds): The Ghrelin System.
Endocr Dev. Basel, Karger, 2013, vol 25, pp 59–68 (DOI: 10.1159/000346054)

Other than Growth Hormone Neuroendocrine Actions of Ghrelin

Andrea Benso · Elisa Calvi · Elena Gramaglia · Ilaria Olivetti · Michela Tomelini · Ezio Ghigo · Fabio Broglio

Department of Medical Sciences, Division of Endocrinology, Diabetology and Metabolism, University of Turin, Turin, Italy

Abstract

Besides its growth hormone-releasing effect, ghrelin has been demonstrated to influence other hormonal systems, such as the hypothalamo-pituitary-adrenal axis, prolactin secretion, the thyroid axis as well as the gonadal axis. Ghrelin and its analogues stimulate the hypothalamo-pituitary-adrenal axis independent of the pituitary, via the hypothalamus, involving both corticotrophin-releasing hormone, arginine-vasopressin and neuropeptide Y stimulation. In adrenocortocotropic hormone (ACTH)-secreting tumors, the ghrelin receptor is pathologically expressed, thus accounting for especially high ACTH and cortisol responses to ghrelin and GH secretagogues in patients with Cushing's disease. Ghrelin stimulates prolactin release most probably from the somatomammotroph cells of the pituitary gland. The effect of ghrelin on the pituitary regulation of the thyroid axis is controversial and its role in the physiological control of thyroid function is still matter of investigation. On the other hand, ghrelin has been reported to exert an inhibitory effect on follicle-stimulating hormone and, in particular, on luteinizing hormone, probably via an inhibitory effect exerted at the hypothalamic level on gonadotropin-releasing hormone secretion.

Before the discovery of ghrelin, many studies in animals and humans had demonstrated that synthetic growth hormone secretagogues (GHS) exert a nonspecific biological effect, acting not only on growth hormone (GH) release but also on the secretion of other pituitary hormones, such as prolactin (PRL) and adrenocorticotropic hormone (ACTH) [1]. As a consequence, since its isolation, ghrelin was deeply investigated not only for its GH-releasing properties but also for its influence on the other hypothalamic-pituitary axes.

Already in the first studies, the potential complexity of the mechanisms underlying the pituitary actions of ghrelin was evident. In fact, the finding of considerable plasma concentrations in healthy humans together with the evidence of the dose dependency of the GH-releasing effect when ghrelin was injected intravenously, clearly suggested that ghrelin, once secreted from the stomach, was able to reach and activate the pituitary [2]. Furthermore, the detection of ghrelin mRNA transcripts in the brain and the localization of ghrelin-immunoreactive neurons in the hypothalamic arcuate nucleus also indicated that ghrelin may directly act on the hypothalamus, where GHS receptor (GHS-R) mRNA is known to be expressed, or be transported to the anterior pituitary gland [2].

Finally, the expression of GHS-R mRNA in peripheral tissues (i.e. thyroid, adrenal, heart, lung, pancreas, spleen, intestine and adipose tissue) further broadened the spectrum of potential ghrelin actions even in peripheral tissues [3].

In this chapter the neuroendocrine effects of ghrelin on the hypothalamo-pituitary-adrenal axis, PRL secretion, the hypothalamo-pituitary-thyroid axis and the hypothalamo-pituitary-gonadal axis are reviewed.

Hypothalamo-Pituitary-Adrenal Axis

The stimulatory effect of several synthetic GHS on the activity of the hypothalamo-pituitary-adrenal axis was observed in different animal models many years before the discovery of ghrelin [1], though considered of minor relevance by the majority of the authors [1]. In particular, the acute administration of GH-releasing peptide (GHRP)-6, GHRP-1, GHRP-2, hexarelin, L-692,429 and MK-0677 was shown to induce a clear stimulatory response on both ACTH and cortisol secretion [1].

A similar stimulatory effect on the hypothalamo-pituitary-adrenal axis was also soon demonstrated for the natural ligand of GHS-R, ghrelin, despite negative preliminary studies [2]. Takaya et al. [4] investigated the endocrine effects of the acute intravenous ghrelin administration in 6 normal male adults. They showed that, along with a strong GH-releasing effect, ghrelin stimulates ACTH and cortisol secretion, in a dose-dependent manner. Accordingly, Arvat et al. [5] reported that the ACTH and cortisol responses to ghrelin administration in humans was higher than that observed after the administration of synthetic GHS, such as hexarelin, the ACTH stimulatory effect of which was already shown to be similar to that observed after naloxone, arginine-vasopressin (AVP) and corticotrophin-releasing hormone (CRH).

Very interestingly, in the same study, Arvat et al. [5] also recorded a significant increase in aldosterone levels after ghrelin but not after hexarelin administration, probably due to the higher ACTH levels achieved by ghrelin injection, though a direct action on the adrenal gland cannot be ruled out, also considering the existence of specific GHS binding sites at this level [6].

More recently, it has been also demonstrated that the central actions of ghrelin include an anxiogenic effect that is abolished by pretreatment with a CRH antagonist in rodents [7]. All this evidence attracted interest about the role of ghrelin in the control of the hypothalamus-pituitary-adrenal axis in physiological and pathophysiological conditions, particularly in Cushing's syndrome.

The ACTH-releasing effect of ghrelin has been shown to be, at least in part, mediated by hypothalamic action, via CRH-, AVP- and neuropeptide Y (NPY)-related mechanisms. In fact, ghrelin has been shown to stimulate CRH and AVP release by the hypothalamus [1, 8, 9]; in particular, the release of CRH by the paraventricular nucleus might involve inhibition of GABAergic neurones, as indicated by both animal and human studies [10, 11]. More recently, Kageyama et al. [12] found that ghrelin stimulates both CRH and AVP mRNA levels in incubated 4B rat hypothalamic cells, suggesting also a direct action of ghrelin at this level.

Moreover, ghrelin has also been shown able to stimulate the release of NPY from rat hypothalamic explants in vitro [9]. In addition, a significant coexpression of GHS-R and NPY mRNA has been shown in the arcuate nucleus, where GHS-R mRNA has been found to be expressed in the 94% of NPY neurons [13]. Accordingly, Wang et al. [14] demonstrated that both intravenous and intraperitoneal injection of ghrelin induce the expression of *c-fos* in the NPY neurons of the hypothalamic arcuate nucleus in rats. Notably, NPY is known to stimulate CRH secretion from rat hypothalamus in vitro and the potassium-evoked AVP release from hypothalamic explants [15]. A central injection of NPY stimulates AVP release in rats also in vivo [16]. Therefore, it is possible that the action of ghrelin on AVP release could be mediated by NPY neurons. Examining the effects of central and systemic administration of ghrelin on AVP release in conscious rats, Ishizaki et al. [17] showed that both intracerebroventricular and intravenous injection of ghrelin stimulates AVP release even at a very low dose, with a quick and long-lasting effect; interestingly, the pretreatment with anti-NPY serum significantly suppressed the ghrelin-induced AVP release [17] further supporting the hypothesis of a functional interrelationship between NPY and AVP.

The central nervous system-mediated action of ghrelin is further supported by the evidence that neither somatostatin nor cortistatin, a neuropeptide with a high structural homology with somatostatin, could affect the ghrelin-induced hypothalamo-pituitary-adrenal axis response [18], in agreement with previous studies with synthetic GHS [19].

Notably, in 2005 ghrelin mRNA was identified in neurons of the rat arcuate nucleus, indicating that ghrelin is locally produced in the hypothalamus, which represents the major source of ghrelin in the central nervous system [20].

Similarly to synthetic GHS, the stimulatory effect of ghrelin on ACTH and cortisol secretion has been shown to be remarkably enhanced, despite hypercortisolism, in pituitary ACTH-dependent Cushing's disease [21]. The stimulatory effect of ghrelin and GHS on corticotroph secretion in this pathological condition is higher than that of CRH, suggesting a particular sensitivity of the tumoral corticotroph cells to these compounds [21], and is generally more marked in patients bearing ACTH-secreting micro- rather than macro-adenoma [22], at least in vivo. This observation was of particular interest considering that, meantime, the GH response to ghrelin and synthetic GHS was found to be reduced in hypercortisolemic patients with Cushing's syndrome as well as in subjects exposed to exogenous glucocorticoids [23].

Although the ACTH-releasing effect of ghrelin and GHS is exclusively mediated at the central level in physiological conditions, its enhancement in the presence of ACTH-secreting tumors is, instead, likely to reflect direct action on the neoplastic tissues [24], also taking into account that the presence of GHS-R mRNA as well as of ghrelin has been found both in normal and adenomatous pituitary [25]. In fact, ghrelin itself has been detected in normal and tumoral corticotrophs, at both mRNA and peptide levels, suggesting an intrapituitary autocrine/paracrine loop [24, 26]. Accordingly, a peculiar ACTH hyperresponsiveness to ghrelin and GHS has been observed also in ectopic ACTH-secreting tumors [27].

More recently, Pecori Giraldi et al. [28] demonstrated that ghrelin is able to directly stimulate ACTH secretion from human pituitary corticotroph cells collected from nine ACTH-secreting pituitary adenomas during trans-sphenoidal surgery. Differently from previous observations in humans in vivo [21, 22], the stimulatory effect of ghrelin described by these authors in vitro was consistently lower than that exerted by CRH [28], suggesting that ghrelin acts on both hypothalamic and pituitary sites to stimulate ACTH secretion in patients with Cushing's disease.

Interestingly, a marked increase of free cytosolic calcium concentration in corticotropinoma cells from patients with Cushing's disease after ghrelin administration has been demonstrated [26]. Furthermore, ghrelin has been shown to be co-stored within ACTH-containing secretory granules, suggesting a potential direct action of ghrelin on neoplastic tissue, likely through an autocrine/paracrine mechanism [26].

Lactotroph Function

According to previous in vitro and in vivo studies on synthetic GHS [1], Takaya et al. [4] first demonstrated that ghrelin administration induces a slight and dose-dependent PRL secretion. Nevertheless, there is a lot of evidence showing no effect in vivo in animal models such as dogs and rats [1]. The species specificity of PRL secretion could be explained by higher levels of mammosomatotroph cells in humans than in animals. In fact, unlike ghrelin-stimulated ACTH release, the PRL secretion seems to be induced by a direct action on this cell type at the pituitary level [4].

Again, similarly to that observed about the hypothalamo-pituitary-adrenal axis, the effect of ghrelin on PRL secretion was significantly higher than that of hexarelin, a synthetic GHS [5].

The influence of the ovarian steroids during the normal menstrual cycle on the pituitary secretion of GH and PRL has been recently studied in 10 women during the different phases of the menstrual cycle [29]. No difference was observed in GH and PRL response to ghrelin among the early follicular, the late follicular and the midluteal phases of the menstrual cycle at all time points, suggesting that the physiological secretion of endogenous ovarian steroids in women does not affect the neuroendocrine action of ghrelin. More interestingly, in the same study, an increased dopaminergic tone, following bromocriptine administration, has been shown able to abolish the stimulatory effect on PRL secretion and to reduce the ghrelin-induced GH increase [29]. Moreover, the stimulating effect of ghrelin on PRL secretion has been shown not to be additive with that of thyrotropin-releasing hormone or of metoclopramide [29].

As previously stated, ghrelin and GHS-R mRNA have been found in normal and adenomatous human pituitary tissue including lactotroph adenomas [25]. At present, there are no data in the literature about the effect of ghrelin administration in prolactinomas; however, previous studies with synthetic GHS demonstrated that these compounds do not induce PRL release in patients with prolactinomas in vivo, though a stimulatory effect has been shown in vitro [1].

Hypothalamo-Pituitary-Thyroid Axis

As fully described in others chapters of this book, ghrelin is an orexigenic factor promoting feeding, adiposity and weight gain also via a decrease of thermogenesis and energy expenditure. On the other hand, thyroid hormones stimulate the metabolic rate of many tissues inducing thermogenesis, energy consumption and weight loss [30]. On the whole, ghrelin actions, leading to a positive energy balance, counteract those of thyroid hormones in the regulation of energy homeostasis, suggesting that ghrelin may exert an inhibitory modulation on the hypothalamo-pituitary-thyroid axis.

In this respect, many studies showed contrasting results. Experiments in rats demonstrated that intracerebroventricular ghrelin administration is able to reduce serum thyroid-stimulating hormone (TSH) levels [31]. Conversely, no significant variation of TSH levels after intravenous ghrelin administration was shown in humans [4].

A recent study determined nocturnal serum levels of free triiodothyronine (fT3), free thyroxine (fT4), TSH, and thyroid-binding globulin in 20 healthy adults after consecutives boluses of acylated ghrelin (50 μg at 22.00, 23.00, 00.00 and 01.00 h) [32]. After ghrelin administration fT4 plasma levels were significantly higher and TSH concentration lower than after placebo. No differences were observed in fT3 and thyroid-binding globulin secretory pattern at any time. The early rise in fT4 levels suggested a direct action of ghrelin on the thyroid gland, where GHS-R was actually identified [33]. Although it could not be excluded that TSH decrease was consequent to a feedback inhibition through fT4, these results could also suggest that ghrelin may directly suppress TSH secretion at the hypothalamic level [32].

In order to better understand the correlation between ghrelin and the recurrent alterations of energy homeostasis in thyroid functional disorders, Caminos and colleagues evaluated plasma ghrelin concentrations and gastric ghrelin mRNA expression in artificially induced hypothyroid and hyperthyroid rats [34]. Their results showed that hypothyroidism condition resulted in a marked increase in gastric ghrelin mRNA as well as in circulating ghrelin plasma levels, while being decreased in hyperthyroid rats [34]. On this evidence they suggested that hypothyroidism leads to a state of resistance in relation to the orexigenic effects of ghrelin, the nature of which is still unclear [34]. In humans, plasma ghrelin levels have been variably reported to be reduced or unaffected in hyperthyroidism and unaffected or increased in hypothyroidism [35, 36]. More recently, Molica et al. [37] investigated ghrelin-induced GH, ACTH and cortisol release in patients with thyrotoxicosis before and after thyreostatic treatment. GH values after ghrelin administration resulted lower in hyperthyroidism, and ACTH response was twofold higher, suggesting that thyroid hormones are likely to affect the neuroendocrine action of ghrelin [37].

Hypothalamo-Pituitary-Gonadal Axis

It is well known that prolonged food deprivation is associated with a reduced reproductive activity [38]. In fact, sufficient energy stores are necessary to achieve pubertal development, growth and fertility. As already mentioned and described in other chapters of this book, ghrelin plays a fundamental role in the regulation of energy homeostasis, stimulating appetite and increasing food intake and adiposity. In addition, increased levels of ghrelin are associated with conditions of fasting and malnutrition (i.e. anorexia nervosa), usually accompanied by amenorrhea and suppressed LH pulsatility. On these bases, ghrelin, as a signal of energy shortage, has been supposed to exert an inhibitory role in the regulation of the hypothalamo-pituitary-gonadal axis.

According to this hypothesis, intracerebroventricular administration of ghrelin during in vivo animal studies in female rats, rhesus monkeys and sheep was able to suppress LH secretion without affecting FSH release and to delay onset of puberty in male rats [39]. In vitro experiments in rodent models showed that ghrelin reduce gonadotropin-releasing hormone (GnRH) secretion from hypothalamic fragments and LH responsiveness to GnRH but directly stimulates LH and FSH secretion by pituitary tissue [39].

The effects of consecutive intravenous ghrelin bolus on the nocturnal secretion patterns of LH and testosterone have also been examined in human males, confirming that ghrelin is able to suppress LH secretion by delaying the next pulse and decreasing its amplitude [39].

As far as FSH secretion is concerned, conflicting results have been reported [4, 39]. In order to evaluate whether ghrelin suppresses FSH secretion in humans, the same authors examined night-time FSH secretion after four 50-μg ghrelin injections in 10 healthy males [39]. Their results demonstrated for the first time that ghrelin is able to reduce both LH and FSH secretion in humans, probably as the consequence of the inhibitory effect on GnRH secretion [39]. Nevertheless, the suppression of FSH was modest and lower than that of LH, confirming that FSH secretion is less dependent on GnRH. More recently, Kluge et al. [40] demonstrated for the first time that ghrelin inhibits FSH and LH secretion also in human females, according to previous evidence in animals and humans [39].

In order to evaluate whether this action is mediated at the pituitary or the hypothalamic level, Lanfranco et al. [41] demonstrated that ghrelin inhibits both spontaneous and naloxone-stimulated LH secretion but does not modify the LH response to GnRH. This evidence suggests that the effect of ghrelin on gonadal function could be mediated by the central nervous system and not directly at the pituitary level. Several potential candidates have been suggested to be the mediator of this action: several orexigenic factors also implicated in the central control of the gonadal axis (i.e. NPY, agouti-related peptide and orexin) but also CRH. In fact, it was shown that ghrelin effect on LH is prevented by a nonselective antagonist of CRH in monkeys [39]. A direct effect of ghrelin on the GnRH pulse generator in the mediobasal hypothalamus, where ghrelin receptor is widely expressed, has also been postulated [41].

Neuroendocrine Actions of the Alternative Ghrelin Gene Products: Unacylated Ghrelin and Obestatin

One of the peculiarities of ghrelin is that the modification by n-octanoic acid, an unprecedented mechanism in mammals, is essential to bind GHS-R1a and to exert its neuroendocrine activities. Nevertheless, the predominant form of ghrelin in serum is the unacylated one; as described elsewhere in this book, unacylated ghrelin (UAG) is not biologically inactive, being able to modulate important metabolic functions and sharing with the acylated form some cardiovascular and antiproliferative actions, in line with the theory of the existence of different receptors subtypes for GHS.

On these bases, our group compared the endocrine activity of acylated ghrelin with that of UAG in healthy volunteers showing that the administration of UAG alone does not induce any change in GH, PRL, ACTH and cortisol levels and does not affect the stimulatory effect of ghrelin on these hormones [42].

Similarly, it has been shown that both intravenous and intracerebroventricular administration of obestatin, another product of ghrelin gene, have not a stimulatory effect on GH, PRL, ACTH, TSH, FSH and LH, at least in rats, despite abundant levels of GPR39 mRNA, an obestatin receptor, have been found on pituitary [43].

More recently, the effects of UAG on gonadotropin secretion in pubertal and adult male rats were examined by Martini et al. [39]. These authors showed that UAG administration is able to reproduce the inhibitory effect of ghrelin in terms of LH secretion and puberty onset, suggesting an action independent from the GHS-R1a pathways and opening new perspectives on ghrelin role in the regulation of gonadotropic function [39].

Conclusions

Besides its GH-releasing effect, ghrelin has been demonstrated to influence other hormonal systems, such as the HPA axis, prolactin secretion, the thyroid axis as well as the gonadal axis. Ghrelin and its analogues stimulate the HPA axis independent of the pituitary, via the hypothalamus, involving CRH, AVP and NPY stimulation. In ACTH-secreting tumors, ghrelin receptor is pathologically expressed, thus accounting for especially high ACTH and cortisol responses to ghrelin and GH secretagogues in patients with Cushing's disease.

Ghrelin stimulates prolactin release most probably from the somatomammotroph cells of the pituitary gland. The effect of ghrelin on the pituitary regulation of the thyroid axis is controversial and its role in the physiological control of thyroid function is still matter of investigation. On the other hand, ghrelin has been reported to exert an inhibitory effect on FSH and, in particular on LH, probably via an inhibitory effect exerted at the hypothalamic levels on GnRH secretion, both via a direct inhibition of the GnRH pulse generator in the mediobasal hypothalamus, and via NPY, agouti-related peptide, orexin and CRH related mechanisms.

References

1 Ghigo E, Arvat E, Broglio F, Giordano R, Gianotti L, Muccioli G, Papotti M, Graziani A, Bisi G, Deghenghi R, Camanni F: Endocrine and non-endocrine activities of growth hormone secretagogues in humans. Horm Res 1999;51(suppl 3):9–15.

2 Kojima M, Hosoda H, Matsuo H, Kangawa K: Ghrelin: discovery of the natural endogenous ligand for the growth hormone secretagogue receptor. Trends Endocrinol Metab 2001;12:118–122.

3 Gnanapavan S, Kola B, Bustin SA, Morris DG, McGee P, Fairclough P, Bhattacharya S, Carpenter R, Grossman AB, Korbonits M: The tissue distribution of the mRNA of ghrelin and subtypes of its receptor, GHS-R, in humans. J Clin Endocrinol Metab 2002;87:2988–2991.

4 Takaya K, Ariyasu H, Kanamoto N, Iwakura H, Yoshimoto A, Harada M, Mori K, Komatsu Y, Usui T, Shimatsu A, Ogawa Y, Hosoda K, Akamizu T, Kojima M, Kangawa K, Nakao K: Ghrelin strongly stimulates growth hormone release in humans. J Clin Endocrinol Metab 2000;85:4908–4911.

5 Arvat E, Maccario M, Di Vito L, Broglio F, Benso A, Gottero C, Papotti M, Muccioli G, Dieguez C, Casanueva FF, Deghenghi R, Camanni F, Ghigo E: Endocrine activities of ghrelin, a natural growth hormone secretagogue (GHS), in humans: comparison and interactions with hexarelin, a nonnatural peptidyl GHS, and GH-releasing hormone. J Clin Endocrinol Metab 2001;86:1169–1174.

6 Papotti M, Ghè C, Cassoni P, Catapano F, Deghenghi R, Ghigo E, Muccioli G: Growth hormone secretagogue binding sites in peripheral human tissues. J Clin Endocrinol Metab 2000;85:3803–3807.

7 Carlini VP, Varas MM, Cragnolini AB, Schiöth HB, Scimonelli TN, de Barioglio SR: Differential role of the hippocampus, amygdala, and dorsal raphe nucleus in regulating feeding, memory, and anxiety-like behavioral responses to ghrelin. Biochem Biophys Res Commun 2004;313:635–641.

8 Mozid AM, Tringali G, Forsling ML, Hendricks MS, Ajodha S, Edwards R, Navarra P, Grossman AB, Korbonits M: Ghrelin is released from rat hypothalamic explants and stimulates corticotrophin-releasing hormone and arginine-vasopressin. Horm Metab Res 2003;35:455–459.

9 Wren AM, Small CJ, Fribbens CV, Neary NM, Ward HL, Seal LJ, Ghatei MA, Bloom SR: The hypothalamic mechanisms of the hypophysiotropic action of ghrelin. Neuroendocrinology 2002;76:316–324.

10 Cowley MA, Smith RG, Diano S, Tschöp M, Pronchuk N, Grove KL, Strasburger CJ, Bidlingmaier M, Esterman M, Heiman ML, Garcia-Segura LM, Nillni EA, Mendez P, Low MJ, Sotonyi P, Friedman JM, Liu H, Pinto S, Colmers WF, Cone RD, Horvath TL: The distribution and mechanism of action of ghrelin in the CNS demonstrates a novel hypothalamic circuit regulating energy homeostasis. Neuron 2003;37:649–661.

11 Arvat E, Maccagno B, Ramunni J, Di Vito L, Gianotti L, Broglio F, Benso A, Deghenghi R, Camanni F, Ghigo E: Effects of dexamethasone and alprazolam, a benzodiazepine, on the stimulatory effect of hexarelin, a synthetic GHRP, on ACTH, cortisol and GH secretion in humans. Neuroendocrinology 1998;67:310–316.
12 Kageyama K, Kumata Y, Akimoto K, Takayasu S, Tamasawa N, Suda T: Ghrelin stimulates corticotropin-releasing factor and vasopressin gene expression in rat hypothalamic 4B cells. Stress 2011;14:520–529.
13 Willesen MG, Kristensen P, Rømer J: Co-localization of growth hormone secretagogue receptor and NPY mRNA in the arcuate nucleus of the rat. Neuroendocrinology 1999;70:306–316.
14 Wang L, Saint-Pierre DH, Taché Y: Peripheral ghrelin selectively increases Fos expression in neuropeptide Y – synthesizing neurons in mouse hypothalamic arcuate nucleus. Neurosci Lett 2002;325:47–51.
15 Korbonits M, Little JA, Forsling ML, Tringali G, Costa A, Navarra P, Trainer PJ, Grossman AB: The effect of growth hormone secretagogues and neuropeptide Y on hypothalamic hormone release from acute rat hypothalamic explants. J Neuroendocrinol 1999;11:521–528.
16 Willoughby JO, Blessing WW: Neuropeptide Y injected into the supraoptic nucleus causes secretion of vasopressin in the unanesthetized rat. Neurosci Lett 1987;75:17–22.
17 Ishizaki S, Murase T, Sugimura Y, Kakiya S, Yokoi H, Tachikawa K, Arima H, Miura Y, Oiso Y: Role of ghrelin in the regulation of vasopressin release in conscious rats. Endocrinology 2002;143:1589–1593.
18 Broglio F, Arvat E, Benso A, Gottero C, Prodam F, Grottoli S, Papotti M, Muccioli G, van der Lely AJ, Deghenghi R, Ghigo E: Endocrine activities of cortistatin-14 and its interaction with GHRH and ghrelin in humans. J Clin Endocrinol Metab 2002;87:3783–3790.
19 Massoud AF, Hindmarsh PC, Brook CG: Interaction of the growth hormone releasing peptide hexarelin with somatostatin. Clin Endocrinol 1997;47:537–547.
20 Mondal MS, Date Y, Yamaguchi H, Toshinai K, Tsuruta T, Kangawa K, Nakazato M: Identification of ghrelin and its receptor in neurons of the rat arcuate nucleus. Regul Pept 2005;126:55–59.
21 Leal-Cerro A, Torres E, Soto A, Dios E, Deghenghi R, Arvat E, Ghigo E, Dieguez C, Casanueva FF: Ghrelin is no longer able to stimulate growth hormone secretion in patients with Cushing's syndrome but instead induces exaggerated corticotrophin and cortisol responses. Neuroendocrinology 2002;76:390–396.
22 Arvat E, Giordano R, Ramunni J, Arnaldi G, Colao A, Deghenghi R, Lombardi G, Mantero F, Camanni F, Ghigo E: Adrenocorticotropin and cortisol hyperresponsiveness to hexarelin in patients with Cushing's disease bearing a pituitary microadenoma, but not in those with macroadenoma. J Clin Endocrinol Metab 1998;83:4207–4211.
23 Giordano R, Picu A, Broglio F, Bonelli L, Baldi M, Berardelli R, Ghigo E, Arvat E: Ghrelin, hypothalamus-pituitary-adrenal (HPA) axis and Cushing's syndrome. Pituitary 2004;7:243–248.
24 Korbonits M, Bustin SA, Kojima M, Jordan S, Adams EF, Lowe DG, Kangawa K, Grossman AB: The expression of the growth hormone secretagogue receptor ligand ghrelin in normal and abnormal human pituitary and other neuroendocrine tumors. J Clin Endocrinol Metab 2001;86:881–887.
25 Korbonits M, Kojima M, Kangawa K, Grossman AB: Presence of ghrelin in normal and adenomatous human pituitary. Endocrine 2001;14:101–104.
26 Martínez-Fuentes AJ, Moreno-Fernández J, Vázquez-Martínez R, Durán-Prado M, de la Riva A, Tena-Sempere M, Diéguez C, Jiménez-Reina L, Webb SM, Pumar A, Leal-Cerro A, Benito-López P, Malagón MM, Castaño JP: Ghrelin is produced by and directly activates corticotrope cells from adrenocorticotropin-secreting adenomas. J Clin Endocrinol Metab 2006;91:2225–2231.
27 Arnaldi G, Mancini T, Kola B, Appolloni G, Freddi S, Concettoni C, Bearzi I, Masini A, Boscaro M, Mantero F: Cyclical Cushing's syndrome in a patient with a bronchial neuroendocrine tumor (typical carcinoid) expressing ghrelin and growth hormone secretagogue receptors. J Clin Endocrinol Metab 2003;88:5834–5840.
28 Pecori Giraldi F, Bucciarelli LG, Saccani A, Scacchi M, Pesce S, Losa M, Cavagnini F: Ghrelin stimulates adrenocorticotrophic hormone (ACTH) secretion by human ACTH-secreting pituitary adenomas in vitro. J Neuroendocrinol 2007;19:208–212.
29 Angelidis G, Dafopoulos K, Messini CI, Valotassiou V, Georgoulias P, Messinis IE: Ghrelin: new insights into female reproductive system-associated disorders and pregnancy. Reprod Sci 2012;19:903–910.
30 Kim B: Thyroid hormone as a determinant of energy expenditure and the basal metabolic rate. Thyroid 2008;18:141–144.
31 Sosić-Jurjević B, Stevanović D, Milosević V, Sekulić M, Starcević V: Central ghrelin affects pituitary-thyroid axis: histomorphological and hormonal study in rats. Neuroendocrinology 2009;89:327–336.
32 Kluge M, Riedl S, Uhr M, Schmidt D, Zhang X, Yassouridis A, Steiger A: Ghrelin affects the hypothalamus-pituitary-thyroid axis in humans by increasing free thyroxine and decreasing TSH in plasma. Eur J Endocrinol 2010;162:1059–1065.

33 Cassoni P, Papotti M, Catapano F, Ghè C, Deghenghi R, Ghigo E, Muccioli G: Specific binding sites for synthetic growth hormone secretagogues in non-tumoral and neoplastic human thyroid tissue. J Endocrinol 2000;165:139–146.
34 Caminos JE, Seoane LM, Tovar SA, Casanueva FF, Dieguez C: Influence of thyroid status and growth hormone deficiency on ghrelin. Eur J Endocrinol 2002;147:159–163.
35 Kosowicz J, Baumann-Antczak A, Ruchała M, Gryczyñska M, Gurgul E, Sowiñski J: Thyroid hormones affect plasma ghrelin and obestatin levels. Horm Metab Res 2011;43:121–125.
36 Gjedde S, Vestergaard ET, Gormsen LC, Riis AL, Rungby J, Møller N, Weeke J, Jørgensen JO: Serum ghrelin levels are increased in hypothyroid patients and become normalized by L-thyroxine treatment. J Clin Endocrinol Metab 2008;93:2277–2280.
37 Molica P, Nascif SO, Correa-Silva SR, de Sá LB, Vieira JG, Lengyel AM: Effects of ghrelin, GH-releasing peptide-6 (GHRP-6) and GHRH on GH, ACTH and cortisol release in hyperthyroidism before and after treatment. Pituitary 2010;13:315–323.
38 Warren MP: Effects of undernutrition on reproductive function in the human. Endocr Rev 1983;4:363–377.
39 Muccioli G, Lorenzi T, Lorenzi M, Ghè C, Arnoletti E, Raso GM, Castellucci M, Gualillo O, Meli R: Beyond the metabolic role of ghrelin: a new player in the regulation of reproductive function. Peptides 2011;32:2514–2521.
40 Kluge M, Schüssler P, Schmidt D, Uhr M, Steiger A: Ghrelin suppresses secretion of luteinizing hormone (LH) and follicle-stimulating hormone (FSH) in women. J Clin Endocrinol Metab 2012;97:448–451.
41 Lanfranco F, Bonelli L, Baldi M, Me E, Broglio F, Ghigo E: Acylated ghrelin inhibits spontaneous luteinizing hormone pulsatility and responsiveness to naloxone but not that to gonadotropin-releasing hormone in young men: evidence for a central inhibitory action of ghrelin on the gonadal axis. J Clin Endocrinol Metab 2008;93:3633–3639.
42 Broglio F, Gottero C, Prodam F, Gauna C, Muccioli G, Papotti M, Abribat T, Van Der Lely AJ, Ghigo E: Non-acylated ghrelin counteracts the metabolic but not the neuroendocrine response to acylated ghrelin in humans. J Clin Endocrinol Metab 2004;89:3062–3065.
43 Yamamoto D, Ikeshita N, Daito R, Herningtyas EH, Toda K, Takahashi K, Iida K, Takahashi Y, Kaji H, Chihara K, Okimura Y: Neither intravenous nor intracerebroventricular administration of obestatin affects the secretion of GH, PRL, TSH and ACTH in rats. Regul Pept 2007;138:141–144.

Andrea Benso, MD, PhD
Department of Medical Sciences, Division of Endocrinology, Diabetology and Metabolism
University of Turin, Città della Salute e della Scienza University Hospital
Corso Dogliotti 14, IT–10126 Turin (Italy)
E-Mail andrea.benso@unito.it

Benso A, Casanueva FF, Ghigo E, Granata A (eds): The Ghrelin System.
Endocr Dev. Basel, Karger, 2013, vol 25, pp 69–82 (DOI: 10.1159/000346055)

Ghrelin, the Gonadal Axis and the Onset of Puberty

Manuel Tena-Sempere

Department of Cell Biology, Physiology and Immunology, University of Córdoba, CIBER Fisiopatología de la Obesidad y Nutrición, Instituto de Salud Carlos III, and Instituto Maimónides de Investigaciones Biomédicas (IMIBIC)/Hospital Universitario Reina Sofia, Córdoba, Spain

Abstract

Puberty onset and reproduction are metabolically gated; conditions of energy insufficiency are associated to perturbations in the timing of puberty and subfertility. The neuroendocrine basis for this phenomenon relies on the regulatory actions of a diversity of nutritional and metabolic cues as well as hormones controlling energy homeostasis at different levels of the reproductive axis. Among these, experimental evidence from different species, including rodents and primates, has accumulated in recent years to strongly suggest that the gut hormone, ghrelin, which operates as signal of energy insufficiency and functional antagonist of leptin, may play a physiological, and eventual pathophysiological role in the regulation of puberty onset and gonadal function. Such a 'reproductive' dimension of ghrelin is likely to include, among others, its ability to modulate gonadotropin secretion, to influence the timing of puberty and to directly regulate gonadal (both testicular and ovarian) functions. In keeping with its proposed role as signal for energy deficit, most of the reported actions of ghrelin upon the reproductive axis appear to be inhibitory, thus suggesting that ghrelin may convey at least part of the suppressive effects of low body fuel stores and energy insufficiency on puberty and fertility.

Metabolic Control of the Reproductive Axis along the Lifespan

Reproduction is essential for the survival and perpetuation of the species, and as such is under the control of sophisticated, and often overlapping, regulatory systems. At the individual level, however, puberty onset and fertility are dispensable. Accordingly, conditions that perturb organism homeostasis, in which indispensable body functions must be prioritized and preserved, commonly result in reproductive impairment. Reproductive maturation and function depend on the proper development and dynamic operation of complex regulatory networks, which integrate upon the so-called hypothalamic-pituitary-gonadal (HPG) or gonadotropic axis [1, 2]. This neurohormonal system is primarily composed by the hypothalamic decapeptide, gonadotropin-releasing hormone (GnRH), the pituitary gonadotropins, LH and FSH, and gonadal hormones of steroid and peptidergic nature [1, 2]. These factors are connected by feed-forward and feedback regulatory loops, which are responsible for the 'core' regulation of the reproductive system [3].

In addition, the precise tuning of the HPG axis involves the regulatory actions of numerous signals. Among those, it is well known that reproductive maturation and function are sensitive to the magnitude of energy reserves and various nutritional and metabolic factors [4, 5]. As a clear example of this phenomenon, critical thresholds of energy (fat) reserves need to be reached in order to attain complete pubertal development and an appropriate reproductive function in adulthood. While this phenomenon is especially relevant in the female, because of the substantial energy drainage of pregnancy and lactation [6], such a tight association is detectable in both sexes, so that conditions of metabolic stress can perturb puberty onset and gonadal function also in the male [7].

Our knowledge of the neurohormonal pathways responsible for the metabolic control of puberty onset and gonadotropic function has considerably enlarged during the last two decades, with the recognition of numerous hormones and central transmitters responsible for the dynamic coupling between energy status, puberty and fertility. A clear example in this front is the adipocyte hormone, leptin, which was recognized more than 15 years ago as an essential neuroendocrine signal linking the magnitude of body fat stores and the reproductive system [4, 5]. Threshold leptin levels are needed to attain puberty and to preserve fertility, suggesting a positive/permissive role of leptin on the gonadotropic axis that is mainly conducted at central hypothalamic levels. However, compelling evidence has now documented that the metabolic-reproductive interplay is multifaceted, so that it includes various excitatory and inhibitory signals, of different sources, acting at different levels of the HPG axis (i.e. at the hypothalamus, pituitary and the gonads) [8]. In this chapter, we will briefly summarize the experimental evidence supporting the contention that ghrelin participates in the metabolic regulation of puberty onset and the HPG axis, with special attention to its sites and mechanisms of action, and its potential physiological, and eventually pathophysiological, relevance.

Ghrelin and the Metabolic Control of Reproduction: General Considerations

As described elsewhere in this book, during the last decade, compelling evidence has been presented supporting an essential role of ghrelin in the control of food intake and energy balance; ghrelin being the only known circulating orexigenic factor [9]. The metabolic dimension of ghrelin is reinforced by the demonstration of its proven role in glucose homeostasis and insulin secretion [10, 11], its central effects on energy expenditure and nutrient partitioning, and its interactions with key signals in energy homeostasis, such as leptin [12]. In addition, solid experimental data has document that ghrelin is a rather pleiotropic molecule, expressed in various tissues, which acts on different regulatory pathways and body functions.

Because of its prominent metabolic role and its proven ability to influence different physiological systems, ghrelin has been proposed as an important neuroendocrine integrator, involved in the metabolic regulation of diverse biological functions. Two important features stress the potential relevance of such a role of ghrelin: (a) the circulating ghrelin levels, mostly of stomach origin, are in most cases negatively correlated with the body mass index [10], and (b) ghrelin has been proposed to operate as long-term signal for energy insufficiency, with reciprocal interactions (in a yin-yang manner) with leptin, as signal of energy abundance [12]. On the basis of these features, evaluation of the roles of ghrelin on the HPG axis became appealing soon after its first identification, in order to define whether, as previously documented for leptin, the gut hormone may function as a putative integrator linking body energy/metabolic status and reproduction. Indeed, the experimental evidence obtained in different species during the last 10 years supports a reproductive facet of ghrelin. As summarized in the following sections, such reproductive roles include regulatory actions at different levels of the gonadotropic axis, and involve also direct expression and functions of ghrelin in the gonads, both in males and females. For the sake of simplicity, we will use the term ghrelin to define the global gene/system and to name the acylated form of the hormone, which is endowed with full biological activity, whereas (when relevant) unacylated ghrelin will be termed by the acronym, UAG.

Ghrelin and the Control of Puberty: Experimental Evidence

Departing from the assumption that ghrelin operates as signal of energy insufficiency, experimental studies addressing its putative role in the control of puberty onset, as the key developmental period highly sensitive to conditions of metabolic stress and negative energy balance [13, 14], have been conducted in rodents. Thus, studies involving acute or repeated administration of ghrelin to pubertal rats do support a function of ghrelin as putative modulator of puberty, with a predominant inhibitory action, in keeping with its observed effects in terms of gonadotropin secretion following acute central administration of this hormone [7, 15]. In detail, repeated injections of ghrelin to male rats during the pubertal transition, at two different dose regimens (low: 0.5 nmol/every 12 h; high: 1.0 nmol/every 12 h), significantly reduced serum LH and testosterone levels, and partially delayed balanopreputial separation, as the external index of puberty onset [16, 17], therefore suggesting a putative inhibitory role of elevated ghrelin levels, as those seen in conditions of energy insufficiency, on pubertal timing in male rodents.

Experimental studies in pubertal rodents suggest also that female puberty, at least in the rat, is less sensitive to the inhibitory effects of ghrelin, as chronic treatment of peripubertal females with low doses of ghrelin (0.5 nmol/12 h for 10 days), similar to those causing delayed preputial separation in males, did not cause major changes in serum levels of gonadotropins or estradiol, neither did it significantly modify the timing of puberty, as estimated by the ages of vaginal opening and first estrus [18]. Notwithstanding, administration of higher doses of ghrelin to female rats during puberty, at a regimen of twice daily injections of 1 nmol ghrelin for 10 days, was able to delay vaginal opening, as well as ovarian follicular development and ovulation in pubertal female rats [14]. As a whole, these experimental studies point out that while both male and female rats are sensitive to the inhibitory actions of high ghrelin levels on puberty onset, males appear to be more sensitive than females. This is opposite to the phenomenon reported previously for leptin; females being more sensitive than males to the regulatory (permissive) effects of leptin in terms of puberty onset [4].

The experimental data on the potential roles of ghrelin in the control of puberty come from rodent studies, while its involvement in the regulation of puberty in order species remains virtually uncharacterized. Of note, hormonal studies have demonstrated a progressive decline in the circulating levels of ghrelin along puberty in humans [19]. Although the functional relevance of such a decline in the pubertal activation of the HPG axis has not been directly addressed, it is tempting to hypothesize that, if ghrelin actually conducts a dominant inhibitory role on puberty onset in humans, such a decrease in its plasma levels, in proper metabolic conditions, would play a permissive role in pubertal onset.

Ghrelin and the Control of the Gonadotropic Axis in Adulthood

In line with the observed effects of ghrelin on the HPG axis at the time of puberty, compelling evidence, coming from various species, strongly suggest that ghrelin is an inhibitory signal for the gonadotropic system in adulthood. Of note, initial studies focusing on the GH releasing ability of ghrelin did not detect overt effects of this hormone on the circulating levels of gonadotropins [20], probably because those analyses were not designed to specifically detect potential changes of the reproductive axis. However, subsequent hormonal analyses, conducted in a diversity of species to address the effects of ghrelin on gonadotropin secretion, have now documented the function of ghrelin as modulator of gonadotropin secretion in mammals. As a whole, the experimental data gathered in the last 7 years demonstrate that, either after systemic or intracerebral administration, ghrelin can induce significant inhibitory responses in terms of LH, and to a much lesser extent FSH, secretion; a phenomenon that is in line with the suppression of gonadotropin levels frequently observed in conditions of negative energy balance [4], in which ghrelin levels are commonly elevated [12].

The ability of ghrelin to inhibit LH secretion in vivo was initially reported in rats, either gonadal-intact or gonadectomized, and was later confirmed in sheep, non-human primates (ovariectomized rhesus monkeys) and humans [16, 21–28]. In rats, the inhibitory actions of ghrelin have been observed in males and females, in adulthood and at earlier stages of postnatal development (see below), both after acute or repeated injection [16–18, 21, 22]. Such an inhibitory effect has been further confirmed in studies addressing the actions of ghrelin at different phases of the ovarian cycle and after gonadectomy [16, 22]. In the same vein, central administration of ghrelin induced a significant reduction of ovarian steroids, estrogen and progesterone, in cyclic female rats [29]. Similarly, chronic administration of ghrelin to adult male rats at undernutrition has been shown to induce a marked drop in serum LH and testosterone levels [30]. Likewise, in the intact sheep and gonadectomized monkey, ghrelin has been shown to suppress different aspects of the pulsatile secretion of LH [23, 24]. Finally, inhibitory effects of ghrelin on LH secretion have been reported also in the human. In detail, two groups have independently described that ghrelin infusion partially inhibits spontaneous LH pulsatility in healthy men [25, 26]. In keeping with this view, negative correlations between ghrelin and LH, FSH, testosterone and estradiol levels have been detected in young male humans suffering from β-thalassemia, a condition linked to perturbations of puberty and gonadotropic function [31]. However, another study failed to demonstrate any significant change in circulating LH levels following injection of a single bolus of ghrelin in healthy cyclic women [32]. This later observation might suggest a sexual-dimorphism in the capacity of ghrelin to suppress the gonadotropic axis, with males being more sensitive than females. In contrast to LH, the effects of ghrelin on FSH secretion in vivo are markedly less pronounced, with predominance of a lack of significant effects in the rat and human. Nonetheless, our group has demonstrated modest inhibitory effects in cyclic female rats at diestrus, following acute intracerebral administration of ghrelin, and in adult male rats, after chronic i.v. infusion of the peptide [16, 17]. In the same vein, it has been reported that ghrelin administration can induce a ~25% reduction in FSH secretion in male humans [33], although the magnitude of such inhibition is much lower than that of LH. Such FSH inhibitory effects of ghrelin have not been replicated in cyclic women [32], suggesting again some sort of sexual dimorphism in the gonadotropin responses to ghrelin in humans. The physiological relevance, if any, of the differential effects of ghrelin on LH and FSH secretion is yet to be elucidated.

Modes and Sites of Action of Ghrelin for the Central Control of Puberty and Gonadotropic Axis

The mechanisms and major sites of action for the regulatory effects of ghrelin on gonadotropin secretion and puberty onset have been explored, although the available information is still fragmentary. Experimental evidence from adult rats strongly suggest that, at least partially, the actions of ghrelin on the gonadotropic axis are conducted at the hypothalamic level, since ghrelin inhibited hypothalamic GnRH secretion by hypothalamic fragments ex vivo [16], and systemic administration of ghrelin caused a subsequent reduction in GnRH pulse frequency by hypothalamic explants in vitro [34]. A similar mechanism might be operative also in pubertal rodents, since the frequency of GnRH pulses was also reduced in immature rats following systemic administration of ghrelin [34]. Whether this central action is conducted directly or indirectly on GnRH neurons is yet to be determined. However, circumstantial evidence suggests an indirect mode of action of ghrelin, since its inhibitory effects on LH secretion in the monkey were inhibited by a non-selective antagonist of corticotrophin-releasing hormone (CRH) [35]. In addition, ghrelin was able to inhibit (at least part of) the stimulatory effects of potent elicitors of gonadotropin secretion acting at central levels, such as kisspeptins (products of *Kiss1* gene) in rats and naloxone in humans [17, 26]. In the same vein, ghrelin has been reported to suppress *Kiss1* gene expression in discrete hypothalamic areas [36]; Kiss1 neurons in the brain being potent excitatory afferents of GnRH neurons [37]. Given the essential roles of kisspeptins as gatekeepers and stimulators of reproductive maturation and gonadotropic function [38], this pathway would provide the basis for, at least part of, the inhibitory effects ghrelin on puberty onset and gonadotropin secretion.

Of note, studies from our group have documented that the inhibitory effects of ghrelin on LH secretion in the rat could be mimicked by similar patterns of administration of the un-acylated for of the hormone, UAG, which strongly suggest that, at least in part, the actions of ghrelin on the gonadotropic axis are conducted through mechanisms independent of the canonical receptor, GHS-R type 1a [17]. Similarly, UAG was as effective as acyl-ghrelin in inducing a partial delay in the timing of puberty both in male and female rats [14, 17]. The physiological implications of this observation are yet to be defined, especially considering the fact that circulating levels of UAG largely exceed those of the acylated hormone. In contrast, despite extensive analyses, we have been unable to identify any significant effect of obestatin, another peptide product of the ghrelin gene, either on LH and FSH secretion (tested at different doses and developmental stages) or in the timing of puberty in rats [our unpubl. data]. As a whole, these observations suggest that the tandem ghrelin/UAG is responsible for conducting the inhibitory effects of the ghrelin system upon the HPG axis, whereas the ghrelin-derived peptide, obestatin, is devoid of any major regulatory action at this level.

Finally, in addition to its central hypothalamic effects, ghrelin can act directly at the pituitary level to modulate gonadotropin secretion [39]. Intriguingly, the actions of ghrelin at the pituitary seem to include both stimulatory and inhibitory effects. Thus, ghrelin has been shown to partially suppress GnRH-induced LH secretion by rat pituitaries in vitro; a mechanism that is likely to contribute to the net inhibitory effect of ghrelin on LH secretion after its systemic administration. However, direct stimulatory effects of ghrelin on LH and FSH secretion at the pituitary have been also described in the rat in different physiologic conditions, such as the various stages of the ovarian cycle and during puberty [22, 39]. Such stimulatory action seems to be opposite (and counterintuitive) with the predominant inhibitory effect of systemic ghrelin in the control of gonadotropin secretion, but it may derive from the differential roles of systemically derived (inhibitory effects) and locally produced (stimulatory actions) ghrelin in regulating gonadotropin secretion. Of note, direct stimulatory effects of ghrelin on LH release have been also described in non-mammals, such as the goldfish [40], but at significantly lower effective doses (pM vs. μM concentrations in the rat). Whether this phenomenon evidences a switch from stimulatory to predominantly inhibitory effects of ghrelin on gonadotropin secretion between non-mammals and mammalian species remains obscure. In any event, it is noted that other prominent biological actions of ghrelin are not fully conserved across evolution; for instance, ghrelin has been shown to inhibit (not to stimulate) food intake in chicks [41].

Ghrelin and Direct Control of the Gonads: Evidence from Expression Studies

As summarized in previous sections, compelling evidence has demonstrated the ability of ghrelin to regulate puberty onset and gonadotropin secretion acting mainly at central levels. Notwithstanding, a number of studies in different mammalian and nonmammalian species have documented the expression and putative direct actions of ghrelin in both male and female gonads. Notably, other factors with key roles in metabolism and body weight homeostasis are also express and/or act directly in the gonads [8, 42–45]. In this section, we summarize the expression data supporting the synthesis of ghrelin and its canonical receptor, GHS-R type 1a, in the testis and the ovary in various species.

Expression of the ghrelin gene and ghrelin immunoreactivity have been demonstrated in the rat and human testes [46–48]. In the mouse, a testis-specific ghrelin gene-derived transcript has been detected, of as yet unknown biological functions [49]. In the same vein, expression of the mRNA encoding the canonical ghrelin receptor, GHS-R type 1a, as well as GHS-R1a immunoreactivity have been reported in rat and human testes [48, 50]. Of note, testicular expression of ghrelin is mostly located under physiological conditions in mature Leydig cells, responsible for androgen production. In contrast, type 1a GHS-R shows a wider pattern of cellular distribution, with detectable expression in Leydig, Sertoli and germ cells; the latter, mainly in pachytene spermatocytes [46–48]. The dynamic nature of the testicular expression of the ligand/receptor tandem is reinforced by the observations, coming from rat studies, that expression of ghrelin in the testis is under the control of pituitary LH, whereas expression of GHS-R is mostly regulated by the ligand, ghrelin, and pituitary FSH [47, 50]. The former is in keeping with the fact that LH receptors are expressed in Leydig cells within the testis, while the latter is compatible with the wider pattern of distribution of GHS-R, which includes also Sertoli cells, which express FSH receptors [1, 2].

Expression of ghrelin gene and ghrelin immunoreactivity has been also demonstrated in rat and human ovaries [51, 52]. In the rat, ovarian expression of ghrelin gene was shown to change across the estrous cycle, with peak levels during the luteal (diestrus) phase [51]. Ghrelin immunoreactivity in rat and human ovaries was mainly confined to young and mature corpora lutea, as well as to interstitial hilus cells, which are also termed Leydig cells of the ovary. No discernible ghrelin signal was detectable in rat ovarian follicles [51, 52]. In the human ovary, GHS-R1a immunoreactivity is detectable in oocytes as well as somatic follicular cells, and luteal cells from young, mature, old and regressing corpora lutea. GHS-R type 1a is also present in interstitial hilus cells and the ovarian surface epithelium [52, 53].

Ghrelin and GHS-R1a immunoreactivity has been reported in human testicular tumors, mainly highly differentiated Leydig cell tumors, and dysgenetic Sertoli cell only tubules [48]. GHS-R1a immunoreactivity has also been described in certain ovarian tumors [53]. However, the role of ghrelin in gonadal tumorigenesis or tumor progression is yet to be defined. In addition, expression of ghrelin and/or its receptor has been reported in the gonads of other mammalian (e.g. porcine ovary [54]) and nonmammalian (e.g. chicken ovary [55] and halibut ovary and testis [56]) species. In pig ovaries, ghrelin immunoreactivity was mostly detected in luteal cells, which is in good agreement with previously reported rat and human expression data.

As final call of caution in this section, it is stressed here that most of the expression studies reviewed above employed analytical tools, such as RT-PCR and immunohistochemistry that do not allow to readily discriminate between expression of the acyl form of ghrelin and other products of the ghrelin gene, such as UAG and obestatin. In fact, some of those expression studies were completed before the recognition of the biological roles of UAG and the existence of obestatin. In this context, it is worthy to mention that analyses using specific antiserum have demonstrated expression obestatin in rat testis, prominently in Leydig cells [57]. In addition, expression of the gene encoding the enzyme responsible for acylation of ghrelin, namely, ghrelin *O*-acyl transferase (GOAT) [58], has been also reported both in the human testis and ovary [58, 59], therefore suggesting that the gonads, which express the ghrelin gene and contains detectable ghrelin immunoreactivity, are capable to synthesize the acyl (and fully active) form of the hormone.

Ghrelin and Direct Control of the Gonads: Evidence from Functional Studies

In line with the reported expression of ghrelin and its functional receptor in the gonads, a number of experimental studies have now documented the ability of this hormone to directly act at the testicular or ovarian level to modulate gonadal function.

The first evidence in the functional front came from rat studies that demonstrated that ghrelin is able to inhibit human choriogonadotropin-stimulated testosterone secretion by testicular tissue ex vivo, and to partially suppress the expression of gene encoding key steroidogenic factors, such as steroidogenic acute regulatory protein, P450scc, 3β-HSD and testis-specific 17β-HSD type III [46]. While, to our knowledge, similar functional studies have not been conducted in humans, ghrelin expression in Leydig cells has been shown to inversely correlate with testosterone levels in men [60]; a phenomenon which is compatible (although do not conclusively prove) with an inhibitory effect of ghrelin also on human testicular steroidogenesis. In addition, in the rat testis, ghrelin is able to inhibit the gene expression of relevant Sertoli cell products, such as stem cell factor, with relevant roles in spermatogenesis and Leydig cell proliferation [61], and suppresses the proliferative activity of immature Leydig cells in rat testis [61]. Given the timed pattern of acquisition of ghrelin expression by Leydig cells during maturation (as only mature Leydig cells express ghrelin), this has been proposed as an autoregulatory factor, which contributes to the cessation of Leydig cell proliferation once a certain degree of cellular maturity, as signaled by local ghrelin expression, is attained [61].

Concerning the ovary, ghrelin has been reported to decrease estradiol and progesterone secretion by cultured human granulosa-lutein cells through a GHS-R1a dependent mechanism [62]. Similarly, progesterone secretion in vitro by human luteal cells is inhibited by ghrelin [63]. In the same vein, ghrelin and GHS-R type 1a are expressed in porcine corpus luteum, where ghrelin inhibits progesterone secretion [64]. Ghrelin affects also the release of luteolytic and luteotropic factors by human luteal cells: it decreases the release of luteotropic factors (VEGF and PGE_2) and stimulates the secretion of luteolytic factors ($PGE_2\alpha$), thus suggesting a putative (predominant) inhibitory role in the control of human luteal function [63]. Of note, human luteal cell functions, including steroidogenesis and the balance of luteotropic/luteolytic factors, are also modulated by UAG and obestatin [65]. Finally, in vitro studies have suggested that ghrelin may influence key relevant ovarian functions in chick, rabbit and porcine species; functions that may include steroid and peptide hormone secretion, proliferative activity and/or apoptosis [55, 66, 67]. Yet, the physiological relevance of those in vitro observations is obscured by the fact that, in some species/conditions, both agonists and antagonists of ghrelin conduct similar ovarian effects.

Ghrelin in Reproductive Disorders: Polycystic Ovarian Syndrome and Hypogonadism

On the basis of its potential role in the control of the HPG axis and gonadal function (see previous sections), alterations of the ghrelin system have been explored in some reproductive pathologies. Considering the physiological roles of ghrelin, those reproductive conditions having also an impact on metabolism have drawn most of the attention in this front.

Among reproductive pathologies, polycystic ovarian syndrome (PCOS) is a complex endocrine disease affecting 5–10% of women at reproductive age. PCOS frequently manifests as menstrual dysfunction and subfertility, together with biochemical and clinical indices of hyperandrogenism [68]. Patients suffering PCOS show also frequent metabolic alterations, including abdominal obesity and insulin resistance. Because of the combined alteration of reproductive and metabolic axes, changes in ghrelin levels have been thoroughly studied in PCOS patients. The majority of the studies published in this area have documented the deregulation of ghrelin secretion in women with PCOS. Thus, fasting ghrelin levels in PCOS patients are disproportionately lower than in healthy weight-matched controls [68–70]. In addition, a negative correlation between hyperandrogenemia and circulating ghrelin has been also observed in PCOS patients [70]. Whether these changes are cause or consequence of the metabolic and endocrine alterations of PCOS remains to be elucidated. In principle, it may be speculated that excess of androgens in PCOS is responsible for the decreased ghrelin levels [71]. Such a reduced ghrelin tone has been related to altered hunger and satiety responses that may contribute to overweight in these patients [68]. In the same vein, because of its function as central inhibitory signal for the gonadotropic axis, decreased ghrelin levels might play a role in the dysregulation of gonadotropin secretion and ovarian hyperstimulation frequently seen in this syndrome. In addition, as yet fragmentary evidence suggested recently that ovarian expression of ghrelin might be altered in patients with PCOS [72], although pathophysiological implications of this phenomenon remain unknown.

Concerning male reproduction, lower ghrelin levels have been reported in hypogonadal men when compared with eugonadal controls [73]; reduction of ghrelin levels may contribute to increased insulin resistance in this condition. In addition, ghrelin may directly regulate spermatogenesis in humans, as ghrelin has been detected in the seminal plasma, although their levels do not significantly differ between normospermic and dyspermic patients [74]. Such direct actions of ghrelin on spermatogenesis in humans are yet to be demonstrated; however, experimental data from rodent models suggest a potential role of ghrelin in the regulation of the seminiferous epithelium in rats [75].

Ghrelin and Reproduction: Conclusions and Open Questions

In the last decade, ghrelin has emerged as an important neuroendocrine integrator, with prominent roles in body weight homeostasis and metabolism, which displays a rather ubiquitous pattern of expression and pleiotropic biological functions. During recent years, evidence has mounted to support a putative role of ghrelin in the control of puberty onset and the HPG axis, acting mainly at central levels. In keeping with its proposed role as a signal of energy deficit, the reproductive actions of ghrelin are mostly inhibitory, thus suggesting that this hormone may contribute to the suppression of reproductive function in conditions of negative energy balance. Nonetheless, experimental data from different species have documented that the actions of ghrelin take place at different levels of the HPG axis, and include not only inhibitory but also some stimulatory effects.

Despite the progress in the area, there are several issues regarding the reproductive dimension of ghrelin that needs further clarification. Just to mention a few examples, the precise pathways and mechanisms whereby ghrelin conducts its inhibitory actions upon the central systems responsible for the control of the gonadotropic axis are yet to be exposed. In this context, the ability of ghrelin to suppress Kiss1 gene expression at the hypothalamus has been documented just by one study in one species; thus, further confirmation of this interesting phenomenon, and whether it translates into detectable changes in kisspeptin expression and/or release, would be desirable. In the same vein, ghrelin has been shown to suppress the secretion of GnRH, but whether this takes place directly on GnRH neurons or involves action on afferents of GnRH neurons other than Kiss neurons should be clarified. On the other hand, the stimulatory effects of ghrelin at the pituitary are intriguing, as they oppose to those of systemic administration of the hormone, but the mechanisms and physiological relevance these pituitary actions remain obscure. Similarly, the basis for the dissociated response to ghrelin between LH and FSH, and eventually in males vs. females, warrants further investigation.

In a related front, a role of ghrelin in the control of other aspects of the reproductive axis, including sexual behaviors, has been recently suggested in experimental models [76], but the physiological importance of such function is yet to be defined. Finally, our understanding of the effects and mechanisms of action of ghrelin in the testis and the ovary in various mammalian and non-mammalian species is still limited and need to be expanded. Likewise, the pathophysiological implications of ghrelin in conditions of altered metabolism and reproductive function have been explored only in some conditions, such as PCOS, but dysregulation of ghrelin secretion may also be involved in other perturbations of the HPG axis associated to metabolic stress, such as anorexia nervosa, cachexia or strenuous exercise.

Acknowledgments

The author is indebted to the members of the research team at the Physiology Section of the University of Cordoba, who actively participated in the generation of the experimental data discussed herein. The work from the author's laboratory summarized in this article was supported by grants BFU 2005–07446, BFU 2008–00984 and BFU2011–25021 (Ministerio de Economía and Competitividad, Spain; covered in part by EU-FEDER funds), grants from the Instituto de Salud Carlos III (Red de Centros RCMN C03/08 and Project PI042082; Ministerio de Sanidad, Spain), and EU research contracts EDEN QLK4-CT-2002–00603 and DEER FP7-ENV-2007–1. CIBER is an initiative of Instituto de Salud Carlos III (Ministerio de Sanidad, Spain).

References

1 Schwartz NB: Neuroendocrine regulation of reproductive cyclicity; in Conn PM, Freeman ME (eds): Neuroendocrinology in Physiology and Medicine. Totowa, Humana Press, 2000, pp 135–146.

2 Tena-Sempere M, Huhtaniemi I: Gonadotropins and gonadotropin receptors; in Fauser BCJM (ed): Reproductive Medicine-Molecular, Cellular and Genetic Fundamentals. New York, Partenon Publishing, 2003, pp 225–244.

3 Fink G: In Conn PM, Freeman ME (eds): Neuroendocrinology in Physiology and Medicine. Totowa, Humana Press, 2000, pp 107–134.

4 Fernandez-Fernandez R, et al: Novel signals for the integration of energy balance and reproduction. Mol Cell Endocrinol 2006;254–255:127–132.

5 Navarro VM, Castellano JM, Garcia-Galiano D, Tena-Sempere M: Neuroendocrine factors in the initiation of puberty. The emergent role of kisspeptin. Rev Endocr Metab Disord 2007;8:11–20.

6 Casanueva FF, Dieguez C: Neuroendocrine regulation and actions of leptin. Front Neuroendocrinol 1999;20:317–363.

7 Tena-Sempere M: Ghrelin as a pleotrophic modulator of gonadal function and reproduction. Nat Clin Pract Endocrinol Metab 2008;4:666–674.

8 Tena-Sempere M: Roles of ghrelin and leptin in the control of reproductive function. Neuroendocrinology 2007;86:229–241.

9 Cummings DE, Overduin J: Gastrointestinal regulation of food intake. J Clin Invest 2007;117:13–23.

10 van der Lely AJ, Tschop M, Heiman ML, Ghigo E: Biological, physiological, pathophysiological, and pharmacological aspects of ghrelin. Endocr Rev 2004;25:426–457.

11 Sun Y, Asnicar M, Smith RG: Central and peripheral roles of ghrelin on glucose homeostasis. Neuroendocrinology 2007;86:215–228.

12 Zigman JM, Elmquist JK: Minireview: From anorexia to obesity – the yin and yang of body weight control. Endocrinology 2003;144:3749–3756.

13 Roa J, Tena-Sempere M: Energy balance and puberty onset: emerging role of central mTOR signaling. Trends Endocrinol Metab 2010;21:519–528.

14 Roa J, et al: Metabolic control of puberty onset: new players, new mechanisms. Mol Cell Endocrinol 2010;324:87–94.

15 Tena-Sempere M: Ghrelin and reproduction: ghrelin as novel regulator of the gonadotropic axis. Vitam Horm 2008;77:285–300.

16 Fernandez-Fernandez R, et al: Effects of ghrelin upon gonadotropin-releasing hormone and gonadotropin secretion in adult female rats: in vivo and in vitro studies. Neuroendocrinology 2005;82:245–255.

17 Martini AC, et al: Comparative analysis of the effects of ghrelin and unacylated ghrelin on luteinizing hormone secretion in male rats. Endocrinology 2006; 147:2374–2382.

18 Fernandez-Fernandez R, et al: Effects of chronic hyperghrelinemia on puberty onset and pregnancy outcome in the rat. Endocrinology 2005;146:3018–3025.

19 Soriano-Guillen L, et al: Ghrelin levels from fetal life through early adulthood: relationship with endocrine and metabolic and anthropometric measures. J Pediatr 2004;144:30–35.

20 Kojima M, et al: Ghrelin is a growth-hormone-releasing acylated peptide from stomach. Nature 1999; 402:656–660.

21 Furuta M, Funabashi T, Kimura F: Intracerebroventricular administration of ghrelin rapidly suppresses pulsatile luteinizing hormone secretion in ovariectomized rats. Biochem Biophys Res Commun 2001; 288:780–785.

22 Fernandez-Fernandez R, Tena-Sempere M, Aguilar E, Pinilla L: Ghrelin effects on gonadotropin secretion in male and female rats. Neurosci Lett 2004;362: 103–107.

23 Vulliemoz NR, et al: Decrease in luteinizing hormone pulse frequency during a five-hour peripheral ghrelin infusion in the ovariectomized rhesus monkey. J Clin Endocrinol Metab 2004;89:5718–5723.

24 Iqbal J, Kurose Y, Canny B, Clarke IJ: Effects of central infusion of ghrelin on food intake and plasma levels of growth hormone, luteinizing hormone, prolactin, and cortisol secretion in sheep. Endocrinology 2006;147:510–519.

25 Kluge M, Schussler P, Uhr M, Yassouridis A, Steiger A: Ghrelin suppresses secretion of luteinizing hormone in humans. J Clin Endocrinol Metab 2007;92: 3202–3205.

26 Lanfranco F, et al: Acylated ghrelin inhibits spontaneous LH pulsatility and responsiveness to naloxone, but not that to GnRH, in young men. Evidence for a central inhibitory action of ghrelin on the gonadal axis. J Clin Endocrinol Metab 2008;93:3633–3639.

27 Harrison JL, Miller DW, Findlay PA, Adam CL: Photoperiod influences the central effects of ghrelin on food intake, GH and LH secretion in sheep. Neuroendocrinology 2008;87:182–192.

28 Lanfranco F, et al: Ghrelin and anterior pituitary function. Front Horm Res 2010;38:206–211.

29 Fang F, et al: Role of ghrelin on estrogen and progesterone secretion in the adult rat ovary during estrous cycle. Syst Biol Reprod Med 2012;58:116–119.

30 Sirotkin AV, et al: Effects of chronic food restriction and treatments with leptin or ghrelin on different reproductive parameters of male rats. Peptides 2008;29:1362–1368.
31 Moshtaghi-Kashanian GR, Razavi F: Ghrelin and leptin levels in relation to puberty and reproductive function in patients with beta-thalassemia. Hormones (Athens) 2009;8:207–213.
32 Messini CI, Dafopoulos K, Chalvatzas N, Georgoulias P, Messinis IE: Effect of ghrelin on gonadotrophin secretion in women during the menstrual cycle. Hum Reprod 2009;24:976–981.
33 Kluge M, Uhr M, Bleninger P, Yassouridis A, Steiger A: Ghrelin suppresses secretion of FSH in males. Clin Endocrinol (Oxf) 2009;70:920–923.
34 Lebrethon MC, et al: Effects of in vivo and in vitro administration of ghrelin, leptin and neuropeptide mediators on pulsatile gonadotrophin-releasing hormone secretion from male rat hypothalamus before and after puberty. J Neuroendocrinol 2007;19:181–188.
35 Vulliemoz NR, Xiao E, Xia-Zhang L, Rivier J, Ferin M: Astressin B, a nonselective corticotropin-releasing hormone receptor antagonist, prevents the inhibitory effect of ghrelin on luteinizing hormone pulse frequency in the ovariectomized rhesus monkey. Endocrinology 2008;149:869–874.
36 Forbes S, Li XF, Kinsey-Jones J, O'Byrne K: Effects of ghrelin on kisspeptin mRNA expression in the hypothalamic medial preoptic area and pulsatile luteinising hormone secretion in the female rat. Neurosci Lett 2009;460:143–147.
37 Roa J, et al: Kisspeptins and the control of gonadotropin secretion in male and female rodents. Peptides 2009;30:57–66.
38 Roa J, Aguilar E, Dieguez C, Pinilla L, Tena-Sempere M: New frontiers in kisspeptin/GPR54 physiology as fundamental gatekeepers of reproductive function. Front Neuroendocrinol 2008;29:48–69.
39 Fernandez-Fernandez R, et al: Direct stimulatory effect of ghrelin on pituitary release of LH through a nitric oxide-dependent mechanism that is modulated by estrogen. Reproduction 2007;133:1223–1232.
40 Unniappan S, Peter RE: In vitro and in vivo effects of ghrelin on luteinizing hormone and growth hormone release in goldfish. Am J Physiol Regul Integr Comp Physiol 2004;286:R1093–R1101.
41 Kaiya H, Miyazato M, Kangawa K, Peter RE, Unniappan S: Ghrelin: a multifunctional hormone in non-mammalian vertebrates. Comp Biochem Physiol A Mol Integr Physiol 2008;149:109–128.
42 Caminos JE, et al: Novel expression and direct effects of adiponectin in the rat testis. Endocrinology 2008;149:3390–3402.
43 Nogueiras R, et al: Novel expression of resistin in rat testis: functional role and regulation by nutritional status and hormonal factors. J Cell Sci 2004;117:3247–3257.
44 Barreiro ML, et al: Pattern of orexin expression and direct biological actions of orexin-A in rat testis. Endocrinology 2005;146:5164–5175.
45 Garcia-Galiano D, et al: Cellular distribution, regulated expression, and functional role of the anorexigenic peptide, NUCB2/nesfatin-1, in the testis. Endocrinology 2012;153:1959–1971.
46 Tena-Sempere M, et al: Novel expression and functional role of ghrelin in rat testis. Endocrinology 2002;143:717–725.
47 Barreiro ML, et al: Cellular location and hormonal regulation of ghrelin expression in rat testis. Biol Reprod 2002;67:1768–1776.
48 Gaytan F, et al: Expression of ghrelin and its functional receptor, the type 1a growth hormone secretagogue receptor, in normal human testis and testicular tumors. J Clin Endocrinol Metab 2004;89:400–409.
49 Tanaka M, Hayashida Y, Nakao N, Nakai N, Nakashima K: Testis-specific and developmentally induced expression of a ghrelin gene-derived transcript that encodes a novel polypeptide in the mouse. Biochim Biophys Acta 2001;1522:62–65.
50 Barreiro ML, et al: Developmental, stage-specific, and hormonally regulated expression of growth hormone secretagogue receptor messenger RNA in rat testis. Biol Reprod 2003;68:1631–1640.
51 Caminos JE, et al: Expression of ghrelin in the cyclic and pregnant rat ovary. Endocrinology 2003;144:1594–1602.
52 Gaytan F, et al: Immunolocalization of ghrelin and its functional receptor, the type 1a growth hormone secretagogue receptor, in the cyclic human ovary. J Clin Endocrinol Metab 2003;88:879–887.
53 Gaytan F, et al: Expression of growth hormone secretagogue receptor type 1a, the functional ghrelin receptor, in human ovarian surface epithelium, mullerian duct derivatives, and ovarian tumors. J Clin Endocrinol Metab 2005;90:1798–1804.
54 Zhang W, Lei Z, Su J, Chen S: Expression of ghrelin in the porcine hypothalamo-pituitary-ovary axis during the estrous cycle. Anim Reprod Sci 2008;109:356–367.
55 Sirotkin AV, et al: Novel expression and functional role of ghrelin in chicken ovary. Mol Cell Endocrinol 2006;257–258:15–25.
56 Manning AJ, et al: Ontogenetic and tissue-specific expression of preproghrelin in the Atlantic halibut, *Hippoglossus hippoglossus* L. J Endocrinol 2008;196:181–192.
57 Dun SL, et al: Distribution and biological activity of obestatin in the rat. J Endocrinol 2006;191:481–489.

58 Yang J, Brown MS, Liang G, Grishin NV, Goldstein JL: Identification of the acyltransferase that octanoylates ghrelin, an appetite-stimulating peptide hormone. Cell 2008;132:387–396.

59 Lim CT, Kola B, Grossman A, Korbonits M: The expression of ghrelin *O*-acyltransferase (GOAT) in human tissues. Endocr J 2011;58:707–710.

60 Ishikawa T, Fujioka H, Ishimura T, Takenaka A, Fujisawa M: Ghrelin expression in human testis and serum testosterone level. J Androl 2007;28:320–324.

61 Barreiro ML, et al: Ghrelin inhibits the proliferative activity of immature Leydig cells in vivo and regulates stem cell factor messenger ribonucleic acid expression in rat testis. Endocrinology 2004;145:4825–4834.

62 Viani I, et al: Ghrelin inhibits steroid biosynthesis by cultured granulosa-lutein cells. J Clin Endocrinol Metab 2008;93:1476–1481.

63 Tropea A, et al: Ghrelin affects the release of luteolytic and luteotropic factors in human luteal cells. J Clin Endocrinol Metab 2007;92:3239–3245.

64 Rak-Mardyla A, Gregoraszczuk EL, Karpeta A, Duda M: Expression of ghrelin and the ghrelin receptor in different stages of porcine corpus luteum development and the inhibitory effects of ghrelin on progesterone secretion, 3-beta-hydroxysteroid dehydrogenase activity and protein expression. Theriogenology 2012;77:1505–1512.

65 Romani F, et al: In vitro effect of unacylated ghrelin and obestatin on human luteal cell function. Fertil Steril 2012;97:991–996.

66 Sirotkin AV, Meszarosova M, Grossmann R, Benco A, Valenzuela F: Effect of inhibitor and activator of ghrelin receptor (GHS-R1a) on porcine ovarian granulosa cell functions. Gen Comp Endocrinol 2011;173:105–110.

67 Sirotkin AV, Rafay J, Kotwica J, Darlak K, Valenzuela F: Role of ghrelin in regulating rabbit ovarian function and the response to LH and IGF-1. Domest Anim Endocrinol 2009;36:162–172.

68 Moran LJ, et al: Ghrelin and measures of satiety are altered in polycystic ovary syndrome but not differentially affected by diet composition. J Clin Endocrinol Metab 2004;89:3337–3344.

69 Schofl C, et al: Circulating ghrelin levels in patients with polycystic ovary syndrome. J Clin Endocrinol Metab 2002;87:4607–4610.

70 Pagotto U, et al: Plasma ghrelin, obesity, and the polycystic ovary syndrome: correlation with insulin resistance and androgen levels. J Clin Endocrinol Metab 2002;87:5625–5629.

71 Gambineri A, et al: Anti-androgen treatment increases circulating ghrelin levels in obese women with polycystic ovary syndrome. J Endocrinol Invest 2003;26:629–634.

72 Komarowska H, et al: Ghrelin ovarian cell expression in patients with polycystic ovary syndrome: an immunohistochemical evaluation. Horm Metab Res 2006;38:783–788.

73 Repaci A, Gambineri A, Pagotto U, Pasquali R: Ghrelin and reproductive disorders. Mol Cell Endocrinol 2011;340:70–79.

74 Panidis D, et al: Serum and seminal plasma ghrelin levels in men with normospermia and dyspermia. Gynecol Endocrinol 2008;24:320–325.

75 Lukaszyk A, et al: Immunohistochemical and hybridocytochemical study on ghrelin signalling in the rat seminiferous epithelium. Folia Histochem Cytobiol 2009;47:415–423.

76 Bertoldi ML, et al: Inhibitory effects of ghrelin on sexual behavior: role of the peptide in the receptivity reduction induced by food restriction in mice. Horm Metab Res 2011;43:494–499.

Manuel Tena-Sempere
Department of Cell Biology, Physiology and Immunology, University of Córdoba
CIBER Fisiopatología de la Obesidad y Nutrición, Instituto de Salud Carlos III, and Instituto Maimónides de Investigaciones Biomédicas (IMIBIC)/Hospital Universitario Reina Sofia
ES–14004 Córdoba (Spain)
E-Mail fi1tesem@uco.es

Benso A, Casanueva FF, Ghigo E, Granata A (eds): The Ghrelin System.
Endocr Dev. Basel, Karger, 2013, vol 25, pp 83–90 (DOI: 10.1159/000346056)

Ghrelin and the Cardiovascular System

Jörgen Isgaard

Laboratory of Experimental Endocrinology, Department of Internal Medicine, Sahlgrenska Academy at the University of Gothenburg, Gothenburg, Sweden

Abstract

Although ghrelin was initially associated with regulation of appetite, the cardiovascular system has also been recognized as a potentially important target for its effects. Moreover, experimental and a limited number of clinical studies suggest a potential role for ghrelin in the treatment of congestive heart failure. So far, reported cardiovascular effects of growth hormone secretagogues and/or ghrelin include lowering of peripheral resistance, either direct at the vascular level and/or by modulating sympathetic nervous activity. Other observed effects indicate possible improvement of contractility and cardioprotective and anti-inflammatory effects both in vivo and in vitro. Taken together, these results offer an interesting perspective on the future where further studies aiming at evaluating a role of growth hormone secretagogues and ghrelin in the treatment of cardiovascular disease are warranted.

Apart from the ability to stimulate GH secretion and to exert regulatory effects on appetite and metabolism, it has become increasingly apparent that growth hormone secretagogues (GHS) (synthetic analogues of ghrelin) and ghrelin have a number of effects on the cardiovascular system. The ghrelin system is present in both vascular and cardiac tissues, where it is implicated in various functions. Ghrelin has been shown to have protective effects by inhibiting apoptosis and to improve left ventricular (LV) function during ischemia-reperfusion (I/R) injury. In rats with congestive heart failure (CHF), ghrelin improves LV dysfunction and attenuates the development of cardiac cachexia. Similarly, in short-term studies, ghrelin improves cardiac function and decreases systemic vascular resistance in patients with chronic CHF In the vasculature, ghrelin exerts vasodilatory effects and possibly anti-inflammatory effects that may be of potential importance for the development of atherosclerosis.

The present article will give an overview of the main cardiovascular actions of GHS and also discuss potential central effects which may have importance for the regulation of vascular tonus. Finally, the potential use of GHS and ghrelin as therapeutic agents in heart failure and related cardiac cachexia will be discussed.

Vasoactive Effects

A well-documented cardiovascular action of GHS is a vasodilatory effect observed in both clinical and experimental studies. For instance, in a study by Kangawa et al. [1], a single injection of ghrelin caused a significant decrease in blood pressure.

Several possible mechanisms for the vasodilatory effect of GHS have been suggested. One of the first studies addressing this subject demonstrated an antagonistic action of ghrelin on the vasoconstrictor effect of endothelin-1 in isolated mammary arteries [2]. Experiments using aortic ring preparations from GH-deficient rats treated with ghrelin showed an increased maximal acetylcholine induced vasorelaxation compared with placebo and this vasodilatory effect was accompanied by an increase in endothelial nitric oxide synthase (eNOS) production [3]. Moreover, the vasoactive effect of ghrelin could be blocked by N(G)-nitro-L-arginine methyl ester, a nonselective NOS inhibitor, adding further support for a nitric oxide dependent pathway. However, the same research group has also reported possible vasodilatory effects independent of nitric oxide mechanisms [4].

Anti-Inflammatory Effects

Apart from vasodilatory effects, ghrelin may also have other vasoactive and anti-inflammatory properties. It has been shown that ghrelin has inhibitory effects on cytokine release and it activates nuclear factor-κβ and mononuclear cell binding in cultured human umbilical vein endothelial cells (HUVEC), which could potentially be important, should GHS be considered as therapeutic agents in conditions with atherosclerosis [5]. Additional evidence for anti-inflammatory effects of ghrelin include the findings that T lymphocytes express both ghrelin and the GHS-R and that ghrelin secretion is increased when the T lymphocytes are activated [6]. This may suggest a modulatory role on the immune system, since ghrelin was also reported to inhibit interleukin-1β, interleukin-6 and tumor necrosis factor-α [6].

A summary of the reported vasoactive effects is shown in figure 1.

Central Effects Associated with Vascular Tonus

Another interesting possible mechanism behind regulation of vascular tonus that has recently been reported is a central effect, involving decreased sympathetic nervous activity and resulting lower arterial pressure, observed after unilateral microinjection of ghrelin into the nucleus of the solitary tract of rats [7]. These findings are in line with a previous report describing decreased mean arterial blood pressure and sympathetic nerve activity after peripheral and central administration of ghrelin to conscious rabbits where arterial pressure and renal sympathetic activity were monitored

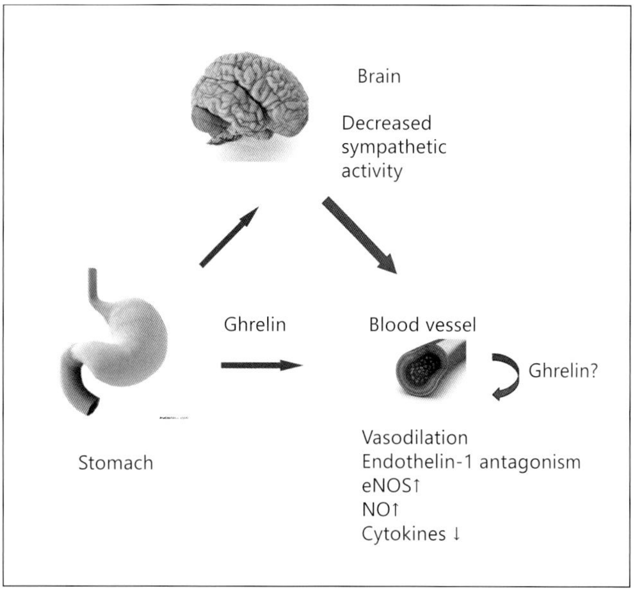

Fig. 1. Possible pathways of interaction between ghrelin, CNS and the vascular system. Exogenous GHS or ghrelin (systemic or locally produced in the cardiovascular system) are likely to interact directly with blood vessels and antagonize the effect of the vasoconstrictor endothelin-1, increase eNOS expression and the production of the vasodilator NO. An alternative pathway may be through the CNS leading to decreased sympathetic nervous activity and an additive vasodilatory effect. Additional vasoactive effects that have been reported include cytokine inhibition.

[8]. The authors suggest that intravenous injection of ghrelin acts, at least in part, on the central nervous system to decrease arterial pressure and renal sympathetic nerve activity, and that central ghrelin is involved in the regulations of the sympathetic nerve activity to the kidney and the baroreceptor reflex in conscious rabbits.

Central actions of endogenous ghrelin have been recently demonstrated in conscious rats treated with a ghrelin receptor antagonist [9]. Mean arterial pressure and heart rate were dose-dependently elevated after subcutaneous administration of the antagonist. Sympathetic blockade of both alpha-adrenoreceptors and beta-1-adrenoreceptors abolished these hemodynamic alterations, suggesting that the increase in arterial pressure and heart rate induced by injection of the ghrelin antagonist are, at least in part, due to the activation of the sympathetic nervous system.

Cardioprotective Effects against Ischemia

Several reports from different research groups using a variety of experimental models indicate cardioprotective effects of GHS against ischemia. In one of the first studies addressing this topic, De Gennaro Colonna et al. [10] used antiserum to GHRH in order to achieve GH deficiency in rats and then treated them with GH or hexarelin for 2 weeks. After killing the rats, their hearts were used for retrograde aortic perfusion under ischemic conditions. As expected, control rats with GH deficiency showed a marked increase in LV end-diastolic pressure (LVEDP) and poor recovery of contractility after reperfusion. In contrast, rats treated with GH or hexarelin had normalized cardiac function. In a further study from the same research group, hypophysectomized rats were pretreated with GH or hexarelin which again protected the hearts from cardiac damage during I/R in vitro [11]. Interestingly, both of these studies suggest GHS effects independent of increased GH secretion since cardiovascular effects of hexarelin were observed in two different models of GHD. An interesting aspect that has been raised is the possibility that cardioprotective effects may not be completely similar, comparing different GHS and ghrelin. Torsello et al. [12] suggested that cardioprotective effects against ischemia after pretreatment with hexarelin could not be replicated by ghrelin. In this study, hypophysectomized rats were pretreated for 7 days with either hexarelin or ghrelin and their hearts were subsequently subjected to ischemia/reperfusion in vitro. During ischemia there was a gradual increase of LVEDP pressure in hearts subjected to ischemia compared to controls. Pretreatment with hexarelin but not ghrelin partially normalized LVEDP and protected the hearts from injury. It could be speculated that this differential effect of hexarelin and ghrelin might in part be due to different affinity to a variety of subtype GHS receptors.

Myocardial stunning is a clinical condition which can be defined as transient myocardial ischemia followed by reperfusion which causes a reversible cardiac dysfunction involving both systolic and diastolic function. A rabbit model was used to study possible protective effects of GH and GHS on myocardial stunning [13]. A significant improvement of diastolic function was observed after pretreatment with GHRP-2, suggesting a novel therapeutic possibility for myocardial stunning.

Several in vitro studies have been performed to explore responsible mechanisms for the protective effect of GHS against I/R. Protective effects of ghrelin and the synthetic secretagogues hexarelin and MK-0677 were tested on isolated perfused rat hearts subjected to I/R [14]. While hexarelin and acylated ghrelin (AG) significantly reduced infarct size, MK-0677 and unacylated ghrelin (UAG) were ineffective. The protein kinase C inhibitor chelerythrine reduced the protection provided by hexarelin. Further evidence for a protective action of ghrelin against cardiac I/R was provided by the study by Chang et al. [15], who showed that administration of ghrelin during reperfusion resulted in improvement in coronary flow, heart rate, LV systolic pressure, and LVEDP, enhanced rates of LV contraction and relaxation and reduced myocardial release of lactate dehydrogenase and myoglobin. These results would suggest not only functional improvement but also protection from tissue injury, which may have important clinical significance.

Proliferative, Antiapoptotic and Metabolic Effects on Cardiomyocytes

Observations of GH-independent effects of GHS have prompted several studies on cultured cardiomyocytes to elucidate possible signaling mechanisms. In studies from our own laboratory, we have found that hexarelin and ghrelin increase thymidine incorporation, indicating increased proliferation of H9c2 cardiomyocytes in a dose-dependent and specific manner [16]. Moreover, binding studies on cardiomyocyte cell membranes revealed specific binding in the absence of detectable expression of the GHS-R1a, which would suggest an alternative binding site in the heart [16].

Possible antiapoptotic effects of GHS have also been studied on primary cardiomyocytes in vitro and cell survival signaling has been described [17]. Both AG and UAG had similar antiapoptotic effects on primary cardiomyocytes, H9c2 cardiomyocytes and endothelial cells with signaling via the MAPK- and PI3K/Akt-dependent pathways [17].

Hexarelin has also been found to decrease apoptosis induced by angiotensin-II in cultured rat cardiomyocytes through inhibition of caspase-3 activity and expression of the proapoptotic protein Bax [18]. Moreover, Bcl-2 expression was increased, providing evidence for antiapoptotic effects of hexarelin through well-established antiapoptotic signaling pathways. Thus, in vitro findings would support both proliferative and antiapoptotic effects of GHS involving well-established cell survival signaling pathways.

Several later reports have further confirmed antiapoptotic effects of ghrelin, independently of the method used to induce cell damage, also in different cell types through similar signaling pathways [19, 20]. Moreover, it has been recently shown that, similarly to H9c2 cells, in HL-1 cardiomyocytes and primary cultured mouse and rat cardiomyocytes, UAG recognizes specific binding sites and both AG and UAG exert antiapoptotic effects [21]. Interestingly, the same study showed that AG and UAG had opposing metabolic effects. Indeed, AG inhibited insulin-induced glucose uptake and had no effect on fatty acid uptake, whereas UAG reversed the AG inhibitory effect on glucose uptake and increased fatty acid uptake and glucose transporter-4 (GLUT4) translocation to the cell membrane [21].

Another potentially important effect of ghrelin on cardiomyocytes was recently reported and involves stimulation of 5′-AMP-activated protein kinase [22]. This kinase has a central role in regulating energy supplies in cells and is activated in hypoxic conditions. Thus, a beneficial effect of ghrelin on cellular energy supply may contribute to the mechanism of cardioprotection.

Experimental and Clinical Use of Ghrelin and GHS in Heart Failure

The various reported cardiovascular effects of GHS prompted studies to evaluate their potential role in the treatment of CHF. In a study from our laboratory, an established experimental approach using ligation of the left coronary artery was used. Intact rats were subjected to experimental myocardial infarction and after four weeks of recovery, the rats were treated with two doses of hexarelin (10 or 100 μg/kg·day, GH 2.5 mg/kg·day) or saline for 2 weeks [23]. Cardiac structure and function were evaluated with echocardiography at baseline and at the end of the experiment. Stroke volume and cardiac output was significantly increased in both the high dose hexarelin group and GH group compared to control rats.

As an alternative method to coronary artery ligation, electric pacing of the heart has been developed as a model for impaired cardiac function. King et al. [24] induced rapid pacing at 240 bpm for 3 weeks in pigs. An orally bioavailable GHS termed CP-424,391 was administered to one group of animals at the initiation of pacing. After 3 weeks of pacing and treatment, GHS-treated pigs had significantly higher fractional shortening and lower wall stress due to cardiac hypertrophy compared to control animals. Serum IGF-1 was increased approximately twofold which would suggest an effect at least partially mediated by an increased GH secretion.

Only a limited number of published studies have so far used ghrelin rather than synthetic GHS to study effects after myocardial injury. Kangawa's group [25] used rats with experimental myocardial infarction and treated them with ghrelin 100 μg daily for 3 weeks. Echocardiography and catheterization were used to evaluate the effects of ghrelin, showing higher cardiac output and fractional shortening in ghrelin treated rats compared to controls.

The experience from clinical trials with GHS and ghrelin in conditions with impaired cardiac function is also very limited at present. A study where 12 patients with CHF were given a single intravenous infusion of human ghrelin or placebo demonstrated beneficial effects in the ghrelin group [26]. Ghrelin significantly increased cardiac index, stroke volume index and decreased systemic vascular resistance within 60 min, all very favorable changes in the condition of CHF. Only one study with longer duration of treatment of patients with CHF has been published so far [27]. In this open study, 10 patients with congestive heart failure of heterogeneous etiology were treated with ghrelin administered intravenously for 3 weeks. Ghrelin significantly increased LVEF, LV mass and decreased LV end-systolic volume. Moreover, ghrelin also increased peak workload and peak oxygen consumption during exercise which would indicate improved systolic function and exercise capacity. There was also a reported decrease in plasma norepinephrine whereas GH increased only transiently after a single ghrelin infusion and did not differ significantly between the groups after 3 weeks of ghrelin treatment. No serious adverse events were observed.

End-stage CHF is sometimes associated with cachexia which is a severe catabolic state characterized by weight loss and muscle wasting. Thus, it is tempting to speculate that ghrelin and GHS may have multiple beneficial effects on this patient population by exerting both positive cardiovascular and orexigenic actions. A recent study using a rat model of heart failure through experimental myocardial infarction demonstrated increased food consumption and weight gain by ghrelin and ghrelin analogues compared to placebo [28]. To date, there are no long-term clinical trials substantiating this hypothesis, although preliminary data suggest that administration of ghrelin increases muscle strength and lean body mass in patients with CHF [27]. It remains to be investigated further if GHS and ghrelin will have a role as therapeutic agents in the treatment of congestive heart failure and more long-term and placebo controlled trials are required. However, the clinical studies published to date certainly open interesting possibilities.

Conclusion

Although GHSs were initially recognized for their GH-releasing properties, it has been recognized that the cardiovascular system is also a potentially important target for GHSs. Moreover, a limited number of studies also indicate cardiovascular effects of ghrelin. So far reported cardiovascular effects of GHS and/or ghrelin include lowering of peripheral resistance, possible improvement of contractility and cardioprotective effects both in vivo and in vitro.

Taken together, these findings would motivate further studies exploring a possible role of GHS and ghrelin in the treatment of cardiovascular disease.

References

1 Nagaya N, Kojima M, Uematsu M, Yamagishi M, Hosoda H, Oya H, Hayashi Y, Kangawa K: Hemodynamic and hormonal effects of human ghrelin in healthy volunteers. Am J Physiol Regul Integr Comp Physiol 2001;280: R1483–R1487.

2 Wiley KE, Davenport AP: Comparison of vasodilators in human internal mammary artery: ghrelin is a potent physiological antagonist of endothelin-1. Br J Pharmacol 2002;136:1146–1152.

3 Shimizu Y, Nagaya N, Teranishi Y, Imazu M, Yamamoto H, Shokawa T, Kangawa K, Kohno N, Yoshizumi M: Ghrelin improves endothelial dysfunction through growth hormone-independent mechanisms in rats. Biochem Biophys Res Commun 2003;310: 830–835.

4 Okumura H, Nagaya N, Enomoto M, Nakagawa E, Oya H, Kangawa K: Vasodilatory effect of ghrelin, an endogenous peptide from the stomach. J Cardiovasc Pharmacol 2002;39:779–783.

5 Li WG, Gavrila D, Liu X, Wang L, Gunnlaugsson S, Stoll LL, McCormick ML, Sigmund CD, Tang C, Weintraub NL: Ghrelin inhibits proinflammatory responses and nuclear factor-kappaB activation in human endothelial cells. Circulation 2004;109:2221–2226.

6 Dixit VD, Schaffer EM, Pyle RS, Collins GD, Sakthivel SK, Palaniappan R, Lillard JW Jr, Taub DD: Ghrelin inhibits leptin and activation-induced proinflammatory cytokine expression by human monocytes and T cells. J Clin Invest 2004;114:57–66.

7 Lin Y, Matsumura K, Fukuhara M, Kagiyama S, Fujii K, Iida M: Ghrelin acts at the nucleus of the solitary tract to decrease arterial pressure in rats. Hypertension 2004;43:977–982.

8 Matsumura K, Tsuchihashi T, Fujii K, Abe I, Lida M: Central ghrelin modulates sympathetic activity in conscious rabbits. Hypertension 2002;40:694–699.

9 Vlasova MA, Jarvinen K, Herzig KH: Cardiovascular effects of ghrelin antagonist in conscious rats. Regul Pept 2009;156:72–76.

10 De Gennaro Colonna V, Rossoni G, Bernareggi M, Muller EE, Berti F: Cardiac ischemia and impairment of vascular endothelium function in hearts from growth hormone-deficient rats: protection by hexarelin. Eur J Pharmacol 1997;334:201–207.

11 Locatelli V, Rossoni G, Schweiger F, Torsello A, De Gennaro Colonna V, Bernareggi M, Deghenghi R, Muller EE, Berti F: Growth hormone-independent cardioprotective effects of hexarelin in the rat. Endocrinology 1999;140:4024–4031.

12 Torsello A, Bresciani E, Rossoni G, Avallone R, Tulipano G, Cocchi D, Bulgarelli I, Deghenghi R, Berti F, Locatelli V: Ghrelin plays a minor role in the physiological control of cardiac function in the rat. Endocrinology 2003;144:1787–1792.

13 Weekers F, Van Herck E, Isgaard J, Van den Berghe G: Pretreatment with growth hormone-releasing peptide-2 directly protects against the diastolic dysfunction of myocardial stunning in an isolated, blood-perfused rabbit heart model. Endocrinology 2000;141:3993–3999.

14 Frascarelli S, Ghelardoni S, Ronca-Testoni S, Zucchi R: Effect of ghrelin and synthetic growth hormone secretagogues in normal and ischemic rat heart. Basic Res Cardiol 2003;98:401–405.

15 Chang L, Ren Y, Liu X, Li WG, Yang J, Geng B, Weintraub NL, Tang C: Protective effects of ghrelin on ischemia/reperfusion injury in the isolated rat heart. J Cardiovasc Pharmacol 2004;43:165–170.

16 Pettersson I, Muccioli G, Granata R, Deghenghi R, Ghigo E, Ohlsson C, Isgaard J: Natural (ghrelin) and synthetic (hexarelin) growth hormone secretagogues stimulate H9c2 cardiomyocyte cell proliferation. J Endocrinol 2002;175:201–209.

17 Baldanzi G, Cutrupi S, Filigheddu N, Cutrupi S, Catapano F, Bonissoni S, Fubini A, Malan D, Baj G, Granata R, Broglio F, Papotti M, Surico N, Bussolino F, Isgaard J, Deghenghi R, Sinigaglia F, Prat M, Muccioli G, Ghigo E, Graziani A: Ghrelin and des-acyl ghrelin inhibit cell death in cardiomyocytes and endothelial cells through Erk-1/2 and PI 3-kinase/akt. J Cell Biol 2002;159:1029–1037.

18 Pang JJ, Xu RK, Xu XB, Cao JM, Ni C, Zhu WL, Asotra K, Chen MC, Chen C: Hexarelin protects rat cardiomyocytes from angiotensin II-induced apoptosis in vitro. Am J Physiol Heart Circ Physiol 2004;286:H1063–H1069.

19 Granata R, Settanni F, Biancone L, Trovato L, Nano R, Bertuzzi F, Destefanis S, Annunziata M, Martinetti M, Catapano F, Ghe C, Isgaard J, Papotti M, Ghigo E, Muccioli G: Acylated and unacylated ghrelin promote proliferation and inhibit apoptosis of pancreatic beta-cells and human islets: involvement of 3′,5′-cyclic adenosine monophosphate/protein kinase A, extracellular signal-regulated kinase 1/2, and phosphatidyl inositol 3-kinase/Akt signaling. Endocrinology 2007;148:512–529.

20 Iglesias MJ, Pineiro R, Blanco M, Gallego R, Dieguez C, Gualillo O, Gonzalez-Juanatey JR, Lago F: Growth hormone releasing peptide (ghrelin) is synthesized and secreted by cardiomyocytes. Cardiovasc Res 2004;62:481–488.

21 Lear PV, Iglesias MJ, Feijoo-Bandin S, Rodriguez-Penas D, Mosquera-Leal A, Garcia-Rua V, Gualillo O, Ghe C, Arnoletti E, Muccioli G, Dieguez C, Gonzalez-Juanatey JR, Lago F: Des-acyl ghrelin has specific binding sites and different metabolic effects from ghrelin in cardiomyocytes. Endocrinology 2010;151:3286–3329.

22 Kola B, Hubina E, Tucci SA, Kirkham TC, Garcia EA, Mitchell SE, Williams LM, Hawley SA, Hardie DG, Grossman AB, Korbonits M: Cannabinoids and ghrelin have both central and peripheral metabolic and cardiac effect via AMP-activated protein kinase. J Biol Chem 2005;280:25196–25201.

23 Tivesten A, Bollano E, Caidahl K, Kujacic V, Sun XY, Hedner T, Hjalmarson A, Bengtsson BA, Isgaard J: The growth hormone secretagogue hexarelin improves cardiac function in rats after experimental myocardial infarction. Endocrinology 2000;141:60–66.

24 King MK, Gay DM, Pan LC, McElmurray JH 3rd, Hendrick JW, Pirie C, Morrison A, Ding C, Mukherjee R, Spinale FG: Treatment with a growth hormone secretagogue in a model of developing heart failure: effects on ventricular and myocyte function. Circulation 2001;103:308–313.

25 Nagaya N, Uematsu M, Kojima M, Ikeda Y, Yoshihara F, Shimizu W, Hosoda H, Hirota Y, Ishida H, Mori H, Kangawa K: Chronic administration of ghrelin improves left ventricular dysfunction and attenuates development of cardiac cachexia in rats with heart failure. Circulation 2001;104:1430–1435.

26 Nagaya N, Miyatake K, Uematsu M, Oya H, Shimizu W, Hosoda H, Kojima M, Nakanishi N, Mori H, Kangawa K: Hemodynamic, renal, and hormonal effects of ghrelin infusion in patients with chronic heart failure. J Clin Endocrinol Metab 2001c;86:5854–5859.

27 Nagaya N, Moriya J, Yasumura Y, Uematsu M, Ono F, Shimizu W, Ueno K, Kitakaze M, Miyatake K, Kangawa K: Effects of ghrelin administration on left ventricular function, exercise capacity, and muscle wasting in patients with chronic heart failure. Circulation 2004;110:3674–3679.

28 Palus S, Schur R, Akashi YJ, Bockmeyer B, Datta R, Halem H, Dong J, Culler MD, Adams V, Anker SD, Springer J: Ghrelin and its analogues, BIM-28131 and BIM-28125, improve body weight and regulate the expression of MuRF-1 and MAFbx in a rat heart failure model. PLoS One 2011;6:e26865.

Jörgen Isgaard, MD, PhD
Dept. of Internal Medicine, Sahlgrenska Academy
Gröna Stråket 8
SE–413 45 Göteborg (Sweden)
E-Mail jorgen.isgaard@medic.gu.se

Benso A, Casanueva FF, Ghigo E, Granata A (eds): The Ghrelin System.
Endocr Dev. Basel, Karger, 2013, vol 25, pp 91–100 (DOI: 10.1159/000346590)

Ghrelin – A Key Pleiotropic Hormone-Regulating Systemic Energy Metabolism

Timo D. Müller · Matthias H. Tschöp

Institute for Diabetes and Obesity, Helmholtz Zentrum München and Department of Medicine, Technische Universität München, Munich, Germany

Abstract

The gastrointestinal peptide hormone ghrelin was discovered in 1999 as the endogenous ligand for the growth hormone secretagogue receptor (GHSR-1a). Since its discovery tremendous research efforts have been directed at unraveling ghrelin's mechanisms of action, revealing that ghrelin is a pleiotropic hormone implicated in myriad of molecular signaling mechanisms. Accordingly, ghrelin is the only known circulating peripheral hormone with the ability to promote a positive energy balance by stimulating food intake while decreasing energy expenditure and body fat utilization. Moreover, beyond its ability to promote the release of growth hormone from the anterior pituitary, ghrelin stimulates gut motility and gastric acid secretion, modulates sleep, taste sensation and behavior, and regulates glucose metabolism. Due to ghrelin's ability to promote body weight gain and adiposity via centrally mediated signaling mechanisms, modulation of the endogenous ghrelin system is considered a promising strategy to treat individuals with pathologically reduced body weight, such as patients with anorexia nervosa or cachexia. The aim of this chapter is to summarize the current knowledge of how ghrelin affects systemic energy metabolism.

Discovery of Ghrelin as the Endogenous Ligand of the Growth Hormone Secretagogue Receptor 1a (GHSR-1a)

In the late 1970s, the pioneering work of Bowers and colleagues led to the generation of a group of synthetic opioid peptide derivates that promoted the release of growth hormone (GH) from the anterior pituitary [1, 2]. The molecules, which Bowers referred to as GH secretagogues (GHSs), were generated by chemical modification of met-enkephalin and gave rise to the generation of a series of potent GH-releasing peptides (GHRPs), such as GHRP-6, GHRP-2, and hexarelin [3]. The mechanism of how these molecules promote the release of GH was distinct from the later discovered GH-releasing hormone (GHRH)/somatostatin pathway and remained elusive until cloning of the GH secretagogue receptor 1 (GHSR-1) from swine pituitary and hypothalamus in 1996 [4]. GHSR-1 was identified as a G protein-coupled receptor predominantly expressed in the pituitary, hippocampus, and hypothalamus [5]. In the arcuate nucleus (ARC), GHSR-1 was co-expressed with neuropeptide Y (NPY) [6] and its activation by GHRP-6 increased c-fos expression in NPY neurons [7]. Together, these data suggested the presence of a yet unknown endogenous ligand for GHSR-1 and indicated that this ligand, beyond its ability to promote the release of GH, might be implicated in the regulation of systemic energy metabolism. Thus, after the discovery of GHSR-1 in 1996, research efforts focused on identifying the endogenous ligand for this receptor. However, it remained unknown until 1999 when Kojima et al. [8] identified the cognate ligand for GHSR-1, which they purified from rat stomach extracts, as the 28 amino acid peptide 'ghrelin'. The name ghrelin originates from 'ghre', the Proto-Indo-European root of the word 'grow' [8]. More than a decade after its discovery, ghrelin is one of the most important peripheral key players in the regulation of systemic energy metabolism. Accordingly, ghrelin is yet the only known circulating peripheral hormone with the ability to promote body weight gain and adiposity through stimulation of food intake while decreasing energy expenditure and body fat utilization [9]. Moreover, beyond its ability to promote the release of GH from the anterior pituitary, ghrelin stimulates gastric acid secretion and gastric motility, influences taste sensation, sleep and behavior, and modulates glucose metabolism via regulation of pancreatic exocrine and endocrine function [10, 11].

Synthesis and Activation of Ghrelin

Ghrelin is predominantly synthesized and secreted by X/A-like cells in the oxyntic glands of the gastric fundus [12, 13]. As the stomach is the major source of ghrelin secretion, plasma levels of ghrelin are substantially decreased in both rats [14–19] and humans [20–29] after bariatric gastrectomy. However, lower amounts of ghrelin-producing cells were also found in the intestine [12], pituitary [30, 31], pancreas [32–34], kidney [33, 35], lung [33, 36] ovaries [33] and brain [33, 37, 38]. Notably, not all human studies report changes in plasma ghrelin concentrations after bariatric gastrectomy [39–41], indicating that other sources of ghrelin secretion can, at least to some extent, compensate for the removal of a portion of the stomach.

Ghrelin is synthesized as a 117 amino acid pre-prohormone and is posttranslationally cleaved into a 28 amino acid peptide. The amino acid sequence is highly conserved between mammals, and rat and mouse ghrelin differ by only two amino acids from the human peptide. To activate its only known receptor, ghrelin requires acylation of its serine 3 residue with an n-octanoic or n-decanoic acid, a post-translational modification that is achieved by the ghrelin *O*-acyltranferase (GOAT) [42, 43] and that is unique in peptide chemistry (fig. 1). The highest level of GOAT expression is found in ghrelin-expressing tissues, such as the pancreas and stomach in humans and

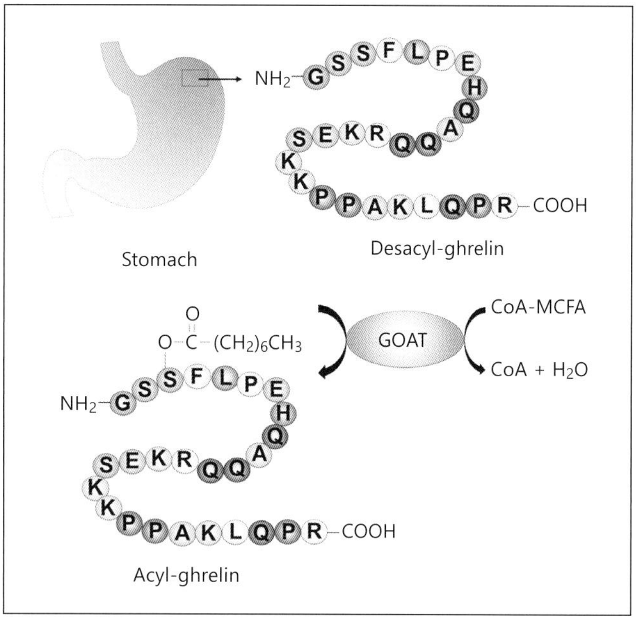

Fig. 1. Posttranslational activation (acylation) of ghrelin by GOAT. MCFA = Medium chain fatty acid; CoA = coenzyme A.

the stomach and intestine in mice [42, 44]. Notably, acyl-ghrelin is absent in mice lacking *Goat,* thus indicating that Goat is the only enzyme activating ghrelin in vivo [43]. The vast majority of ghrelin's metabolic effects, including the modulation of GH release from the anterior pituitary and the regulation of energy metabolism via hypothalamic neurocircuitries, are mediated by GHSR-1, and thus depend on the n-octanoylation of serine 3. However, only 10–20% of circulating ghrelin is acylated and, even though no receptor for des-acyl ghrelin has been identified, several studies suggest that des-acyl ghrelin promotes differentiation and fusion in C2C12 skeletal muscle cells [45], has a cardioprotective effect on endothelial cells and cardiomyocytes [46, 47], and might have some GHSR-1 independent effects on energy and glucose metabolism [48–50].

Ghrelin-Mediated Regulation of Food Intake and Energy Metabolism

Several forms of ghrelin (octanoyl-, desacyl, (nonoctanoyl) acyl-ghrelin) can be found in the circulation and most available immunoassays do not sufficiently disclose to which of those ghrelin analogues they are binding and to what extent they are cross-reacting with other ghrelin-related peptides, e.g. motilin. It is likely that most assays measure total ghrelin-like immunoreactivity including desacyl ghrelin, which accounts for up to 90% of total ghrelin in the circulation. Nevertheless, plasma levels of ghrelin are generally negatively correlated with body weight and increase in response to fasting with a subsequent decrease upon refeeding [9, 51, 52]. Plasma concentrations of ghrelin are typically lower in obese compared lean individuals [53–55] and are elevated in individuals with pathologically reduced body weight, such as patients with anorexia nervosa [56–58], as well as in patients with cachexia associated with chronic heart failure [59, 60], renal failure [61, 62], chronic obstructive pulmonary disease [63, 64] and various forms of cancer [65–67].

Secreted into the circulation in response to fasting, ghrelin was long considered to be a 'hunger' hormone that signals the gastrointestinal fuel status from the periphery to the CNS in order to adjust energy balance through centrally regulated signaling mechanisms. The role of ghrelin as a 'hunger' hormone was supported by the observation that plasma levels of ghrelin follow a circadian rhythm with a preprandial rise, which peaks directly at meal initiation, followed by a postprandial decrease to baseline levels within the first hour after a meal [51, 52, 68]. Current opinion questions whether ghrelin is a 'hunger' hormone, as more recent studies suggest that ghrelin acts more as a nutrient sensor, preparing the CNS for incoming nutrients. This nutrient sensor role of ghrelin is based on the observation that the acyl side chain necessary for ghrelin activation can originate directly from dietary lipids [69]. In line with this observation, mice that overexpress GOAT/ghrelin show increased energy expenditure compared to wild-type control mice when fed with a diet enriched with non-naturally occurring medium-chain triglycerides (MCT diet) [69]. Moreover, in line with its role as a nutrient sensor, ghrelin, independent of its effect on food intake, promotes lipogenesis in white adipose tissue via direct control of the hypothalamic melanocortinergic system [70].

Both peripheral and central administration of ghrelin potently promotes body weight gain and adiposity through a stimulation of food intake while decreasing energy expenditure and body fat utilization [9]. The orexigenic effect of ghrelin is thereby achieved through centrally regulated signaling mechanisms. In the ARC, GHSR1a is co-expressed with Npy and agouti-related peptide (AgRP). Both are anabolic neuropeptides that potently stimulate food intake while decreasing energy expenditure [71]. Accordingly, ghrelin-mediated activation of GHSR1a entails an increased expression and release of Npy and AgRP in the ARC, which, in turn, leads to the activation of anabolic downstream pathways that ultimately results in the stimulation of food intake and a decrease of energy expenditure [72, 73]. Inhibition of AgRP/Npy neurons diminishes ghrelin's effect on food intake, thus indicating that the orexigenic effect of ghrelin is mainly mediated through the hypothalamic melanocortinergic system [74].

Independent from its effect on food intake and energy expenditure, ghrelin stimulates the expression of genes related to lipogenesis in white adipose tissue, such as lipoprotein lipase, acetyl-CoA carboxylase-α, fatty acid synthase, and stearoyl-CoA desaturase-1 [75]. Moreover, in brown adipose tissue, ghrelin decreases the expression of thermogenesis-related genes, such as the uncoupling proteins 1 and 3, an effect that is most likely mediated by ghrelin's ability to decrease the activity of the sympathetic nervous system [75]. In summary, the endogenous GOAT/ghrelin system plays a key role in the neuroendocrine regulation of systemic energy metabolism, and modulation of the endogenous ghrelin system is considered as a promising strategy for the treatment of individuals with pathologically reduced body weight such as patients with anorexia or cachexia.

Ghrelin in the Treatment of Eating/Wasting Disorders and Cachexia

Cachexia (Greek: kakós – bad; hexis – condition) is a multifactorial syndrome characterized by an involuntarily loss of skeletal muscle and adipose tissue mass as a result of a chronic excess of catabolic over anabolic processes [76–78]. Cachexia often occurs in the advanced stages of life-threatening diseases, such as chronic heart failure, chronic obstructive pulmonary disease, end-stage renal disease, sepsis, AIDS and cancer [77, 79]. Patients with cachexia typically have a poor quality of life, poor prognosis, lower response to drug treatment and an increased mortality rate compared to patients without cachexia [76, 80]. Cachexia is often, but not necessarily, accompanied by a loss of the desire to eat (anorexia) and is believed to be the immediate cause of 10–20% of all deaths in cancer patients [80].

Anorexia Nervosa
Anorexia nervosa (AN) is an eating disorder that is characterized by an abnormal eating behavior with disturbances of attitudes towards body weight and shape [81]. Plasma concentrations of ghrelin are typically elevated in patients with AN [56–58], especially in the acute phase of the disease, and rapidly decline when body weight increases during therapeutic intervention [82–84]. Plasma levels of acyl-ghrelin are likewise elevated in patients with AN [56, 58], even when compared to BMI-matched lean women [57, 85]. This indicates that impaired ghrelin sensitivity due to persistent hyperghrelinemia might play a role in the pathogenesis of AN, similar to the frequently reported leptin resistance in obese individuals [78]. Several human studies have assessed the orexigenic effect of ghrelin and its analogs and confirm that ghrelin promotes food intake and adiposity in both healthy individuals [86–88] and patients with AN [89]. Notably, these studies report no adverse side effects of ghrelin treatment.

Cachexia
Plasma levels of ghrelin are typically elevated in patients with cachexia associated with chronic heart failure [59, 60], renal failure [61, 62], chronic obstructive pulmonary disease [63, 90] and cancer [66, 67]. The hyperghrelinemia in these patients might be a compensatory mechanism to counteract the excessive loss of skeletal muscle and adipose tissue mass. Animal studies generally support the potential of ghrelin and its analogs to promote food intake and adiposity in cachexia associated with heart failure [91–94], chronic kidney disease [95] and cancer [96–98]. In line with these reports,

several human studies report a positive effect of ghrelin on appetite and body mass in patients with cachexia associated with renal failure [99, 100], chronic heart failure [101], chronic obstructive pulmonary disease [102], and cancer [103]. Notably, these studies support the safety and tolerability of ghrelin treatment and no adverse side effects have so far been reported [103, 104].

In summary, the endogenous ghrelin system plays a key role in the neuroendocrine regulation of systemic energy metabolism, and modulation of the GOAT/ghrelin system is a promising strategy for the treatment of pathologically reduced body weight and tissue wasting, the key clinical feature of cachexia. However, further studies in larger populations are necessary to clarify the long-term effects of ghrelin treatment and to assess the possible impact of ghrelin and ghrelin-induced growth factor release on tumor growth and carcinogenesis.

References

1 Bowers CY, Momany F, Reynolds GA, Chang D, Hong A, et al: Structure-activity relationships of a synthetic pentapeptide that specifically releases growth hormone in vitro. Endocrinology 1980;106:663–667.

2 Momany FA, Bowers CY, Reynolds GA, Chang D, Hong A, et al: Design, synthesis, and biological activity of peptides which release growth hormone in vitro. Endocrinology 1981;108:31–39.

3 Smith RG, Van der Ploeg LH, Howard AD, Feighner SD, Cheng K, et al: Peptidomimetic regulation of growth hormone secretion. Endocr Rev 1997;18:621–645.

4 Howard AD, Feighner SD, Cully DF, Arena JP, Liberator PA, et al: A receptor in pituitary and hypothalamus that functions in growth hormone release. Science 1996;273:974–977.

5 Guan XM, Yu H, Palyha OC, McKee KK, Feighner SD, et al: Distribution of mRNA encoding the growth hormone secretagogue receptor in brain and peripheral tissues. Brain Res Mol Brain Res 1997;48:23–29.

6 Willesen MG, Kristensen P, Romer J: Co-localization of growth hormone secretagogue receptor and NPY mRNA in the arcuate nucleus of the rat. Neuroendocrinology 1999;70:306–316.

7 Dickson SL, Luckman SM: Induction of c-fos messenger ribonucleic acid in neuropeptide Y and growth hormone (GH)-releasing factor neurons in the rat arcuate nucleus following systemic injection of the GH secretagogue, GH-releasing peptide-6. Endocrinology 1997;138:771–777.

8 Kojima M, Hosoda H, Date Y, Nakazato M, Matsuo H, et al: Ghrelin is a growth-hormone-releasing acylated peptide from stomach. Nature 1999;402:656–660.

9 Tschop M, Smiley DL, Heiman ML: Ghrelin induces adiposity in rodents. Nature 2000;407:908–913.

10 Kojima M, Kangawa K: Structure and function of ghrelin. Results Probl Cell Differ 2008;46:89–115.

11 van der Lely AJ, Tschop M, Heiman ML, Ghigo E: Biological, physiological, pathophysiological, and pharmacological aspects of ghrelin. Endocr Rev 2004;25:426–457.

12 Sakata I, Nakamura K, Yamazaki M, Matsubara M, Hayashi Y, et al: Ghrelin-producing cells exist as two types of cells, closed- and opened-type cells, in the rat gastrointestinal tract. Peptides 2002;23:531–536.

13 Date Y, Kojima M, Hosoda H, Sawaguchi A, Mondal MS, et al: Ghrelin, a novel growth hormone-releasing acylated peptide, is synthesized in a distinct endocrine cell type in the gastrointestinal tracts of rats and humans. Endocrinology 2002;141:4255–4261.

14 Masuda T, Ohta M, Hirashita T, Kawano Y, Eguchi H, et al: A comparative study of gastric banding and sleeve gastrectomy in an obese diabetic rat model. Obes Surg 2011;21:1774–1780.

15 Cummings BP, Bettaieb A, Graham JL, Stanhope KL, Kowala M, et al: Vertical sleeve gastrectomy improves glucose and lipid metabolism and delays diabetes onset in UCD-T2DM rats. Endocrinology 2012;153:3620–3632.

16 Yan L, Zhu Z, Wu D, Zhou Q, Wu Y: Effects of sleeve gastrectomy surgery with modified jejunoileal bypass on body weight, food intake and metabolic hormone levels of rats. J Huazhong Univ Sci Technolog Med Sci 2011;31:784–788.

17 Wang Y, Yan L, Jin Z, Xin X: Effects of sleeve gastrectomy in neonatally streptozotocin-induced diabetic rats. PLoS One 2011;6:e16383.

18 Li F, Zhang G, Liang J, Ding X, Cheng Z, et al: Sleeve gastrectomy provides a better control of diabetes by decreasing ghrelin in the diabetic Goto-Kakizaki rats. J Gastrointest Surg 2009;13:2302–2308.
19 Wang Y, Liu J: Plasma ghrelin modulation in gastric band operation and sleeve gastrectomy. Obes Surg 2009;19:357–362.
20 Leonetti F, Silecchia G, Iacobellis G, Ribaudo MC, Zappaterreno A, et al: Different plasma ghrelin levels after laparoscopic gastric bypass and adjustable gastric banding in morbid obese subjects. J Clin Endocrinol Metab 2003;88:4227–4231.
21 Ariyasu H, Takaya K, Tagami T, Ogawa Y, Hosoda K, et al: Stomach is a major source of circulating ghrelin, and feeding state determines plasma ghrelin-like immunoreactivity levels in humans. J Clin Endocrinol Metab 2001;86:4753–4758.
22 Bohdjalian A, Langer FB, Shakeri-Leidenmuhler S, Gfrerer L, Ludvik B, et al: Sleeve gastrectomy as sole and definitive bariatric procedure: 5-year results for weight loss and ghrelin. Obes Surg 2010;20:535–540.
23 Goitein D, Lederfein D, Tzioni R, Berkenstadt H, Venturero M, et al: Mapping of ghrelin gene expression and cell distribution in the stomach of morbidly obese patients – a possible guide for efficient sleeve gastrectomy construction. Obes Surg 2012;22:617–622.
24 Karamanakos SN, Vagenas K, Kalfarentzos F, Alexandrides TK: Weight loss, appetite suppression, and changes in fasting and postprandial ghrelin and peptide-YY levels after Roux-en-Y gastric bypass and sleeve gastrectomy: a prospective, double blind study. Ann Surg 2008;247:401–407.
25 Langer FB, Reza Hoda MA, Bohdjalian A, Felberbauer FX, Zacherl J, et al: Sleeve gastrectomy and gastric banding: effects on plasma ghrelin levels. Obes Surg 2005;15:1024–1029.
26 Peterli R, Steinert RE, Woelnerhanssen B, Peters T, Christoffel-Courtin C, et al: Metabolic and hormonal changes after laparoscopic Roux-en-Y gastric bypass and sleeve gastrectomy: a randomized, prospective trial. Obes Surg 2012;22:740–748.
27 Ramon JM, Salvans S, Crous X, Puig S, Goday A, et al: Effect of Roux-en-Y gastric bypass vs. sleeve gastrectomy on glucose and gut hormones: a prospective randomised trial. J Gastrointest Surg 2012;16: 1116–1122.
28 Lee WJ, Chen CY, Chong K, Lee YC, Chen SC, et al: Changes in postprandial gut hormones after metabolic surgery: a comparison of gastric bypass and sleeve gastrectomy. Surg Obes Relat Dis 2011;7:683–690.
29 Basso N, Capoccia D, Rizzello M, Abbatini F, Mariani P, et al: First-phase insulin secretion, insulin sensitivity, ghrelin, GLP-1, and PYY changes 72 h after sleeve gastrectomy in obese diabetic patients: the gastric hypothesis. Surg Endosc 2011;25:3540–3550.
30 Korbonits M, Kojima M, Kangawa K, Grossman AB: Presence of ghrelin in normal and adenomatous human pituitary. Endocrine 2001;14:101–104.
31 Korbonits M, Bustin SA, Kojima M, Jordan S, Adams EF, et al: The expression of the growth hormone secretagogue receptor ligand ghrelin in normal and abnormal human pituitary and other neuroendocrine tumors. J Clin Endocrinol Metab 2001;86:881–887.
32 Prado CL, Pugh-Bernard AE, Elghazi L, Sosa-Pineda B, Sussel L: Ghrelin cells replace insulin-producing beta cells in two mouse models of pancreas development. Proc Natl Acad Sci USA 2004;101:2924–2929.
33 Ueberberg B, Unger N, Saeger W, Mann K, Petersenn S: Expression of ghrelin and its receptor in human tissues. Horm Metab Res 2009;41:814–821.
34 Volante M, Allia E, Gugliotta P, Funaro A, Broglio F, et al: Expression of ghrelin and of the GH secretagogue receptor by pancreatic islet cells and related endocrine tumors. J Clin Endocrinol Metab 2002;87: 1300–1308.
35 Volante M, Allia E, Fulcheri E, Cassoni P, Ghigo E, et al: Ghrelin in fetal thyroid and follicular tumors and cell lines: expression and effects on tumor growth. Am J Pathol 2003;162:645–654.
36 Volante M, Fulcheri E, Allia E, Cerrato M, Pucci A, et al: Ghrelin expression in fetal, infant, and adult human lung. J Histochem Cytochem 2002;50:1013–1021.
37 Cowley MA, Smith RG, Diano S, Tschop M, Pronchuk N, et al: The distribution and mechanism of action of ghrelin in the CNS demonstrates a novel hypothalamic circuit regulating energy homeostasis. Neuron 2003;37:649–661.
38 Hou Z, Miao Y, Gao L, Pan H, Zhu S: Ghrelin-containing neuron in cerebral cortex and hypothalamus linked with the DVC of brainstem in rat. Regul Pept 2006;134:126–131.
39 Brinckerhoff TZ, Bondada S, Lewis CE, French SW, Deugarte DA: Metabolic effects of sleeve gastrectomy in female rat model of diet-induced obesity. Surg Obes Relat Dis 2011.
40 Patrikakos P, Toutouzas KG, Gazouli M, Perrea D, Menenakos E, et al: Long-term plasma ghrelin and leptin modulation after sleeve gastrectomy in Wistar rats in comparison with gastric tissue ghrelin expression. Obes Surg 2011;21:1432–1437.
41 Lopez PP, Nicholson SE, Burkhardt GE, Johnson RA, Johnson FK: Development of a sleeve gastrectomy weight loss model in obese Zucker rats. J Surg Res 2009;157:243–250.
42 Gutierrez JA, Solenberg PJ, Perkins DR, Willency JA, Knierman MD, et al: Ghrelin octanoylation mediated by an orphan lipid transferase. Proc Natl Acad Sci USA 2008;105:6320–6325.

43 Yang J, Zhao TJ, Goldstein JL, Brown MS: Inhibition of ghrelin *O*-acyltransferase (GOAT) by octanoylated pentapeptides. Proc Natl Acad Sci USA 2008;105:10750–10755.
44 Sakata I, Yang J, Lee CE, Osborne-Lawrence S, Rovinsky SA, et al: Colocalization of ghrelin *O*-acyltransferase and ghrelin in gastric mucosal cells. Am J Physiol Endocrinol Metab 2009;297:E134–E141.
45 Filigheddu N, Gnocchi VF, Coscia M, Cappelli M, Porporato PE, et al: Ghrelin and des-acyl ghrelin promote differentiation and fusion of C2C12 skeletal muscle cells. Mol Biol Cell 2007;18:986–994.
46 Li L, Zhang LK, Pang YZ, Pan CS, Qi YF, et al: Cardioprotective effects of ghrelin and des-octanoyl ghrelin on myocardial injury induced by isoproterenol in rats. Acta Pharmacol Sin 2006;27:527–535.
47 Baldanzi G, Filigheddu N, Cutrupi S, Catapano F, Bonissoni S, et al: Ghrelin and des-acyl ghrelin inhibit cell death in cardiomyocytes and endothelial cells through ERK1/2 and PI 3-kinase/AKT. J Cell Biol 2002;159:1029–1037.
48 Thompson NM, Gill DA, Davies R, Loveridge N, Houston PA, et al: Ghrelin and des-octanoyl ghrelin promote adipogenesis directly in vivo by a mechanism independent of the type 1a growth hormone secretagogue receptor. Endocrinology 2004;145:234–242.
49 Toshinai K, Yamaguchi H, Sun Y, Smith RG, Yamanaka A, et al: Des-acyl ghrelin induces food intake by a mechanism independent of the growth hormone secretagogue receptor. Endocrinology 2006;147:2306–2314.
50 Zhang W, Chai B, Li JY, Wang H, Mulholland MW: Effect of des-acyl ghrelin on adiposity and glucose metabolism. Endocrinology 2008;149:4710–4716.
51 Cummings DE, Purnell JQ, Frayo RS, Schmidova K, Wisse BE, et al: A preprandial rise in plasma ghrelin levels suggests a role in meal initiation in humans. Diabetes 2001;50:1714–1719.
52 Tschop M, Wawarta R, Riepl RL, Friedrich S, Bidlingmaier M, et al: Post-prandial decrease of circulating human ghrelin levels. J Endocrinol Invest 2001;24:RC19–RC21.
53 Hansen TK, Dall R, Hosoda H, Kojima M, Kangawa K, et al: Weight loss increases circulating levels of ghrelin in human obesity. Clin Endocrinol (Oxf) 2002;56:203–206.
54 Shiiya T, Nakazato M, Mizuta M, Date Y, Mondal MS, et al: Plasma ghrelin levels in lean and obese humans and the effect of glucose on ghrelin secretion. J Clin Endocrinol Metab 2002;87:240–244.
55 Tschop M, Weyer C, Tataranni PA, Devanarayan V, Ravussin E, et al: Circulating ghrelin levels are decreased in human obesity. Diabetes 2001;50:707–709.
56 Nakai Y, Hosoda H, Nin K, Ooya C, Hayashi H, et al: Short-term secretory regulation of the active form of ghrelin and total ghrelin during an oral glucose tolerance test in patients with anorexia nervosa. Eur J Endocrinol 2004;150:913–914.
57 Tolle V, Kadem M, Bluet-Pajot MT, Frere D, Foulon C, et al: Balance in ghrelin and leptin plasma levels in anorexia nervosa patients and constitutionally thin women. J Clin Endocrinol Metab 2003;88:109–116.
58 Harada T, Nakahara T, Yasuhara D, Kojima S, Sagiyama K, et al: Obestatin, acyl ghrelin, and des-acyl ghrelin responses to an oral glucose tolerance test in the restricting type of anorexia nervosa. Biol Psychiatry 2008;63:245–247.
59 Nagaya N, Uematsu M, Kojima M, Date Y, Nakazato M, et al: Elevated circulating level of ghrelin in cachexia associated with chronic heart failure: relationships between ghrelin and anabolic/catabolic factors. Circulation 2001;104:2034–2038.
60 Xin X, Ren AJ, Zheng X, Qin YW, Zhao XX, et al: Disturbance of circulating ghrelin and obestatin in chronic heart failure patients especially in those with cachexia. Peptides 2009;30:2281–2285.
61 Yoshimoto A, Mori K, Sugawara A, Mukoyama M, Yahata K, et al: Plasma ghrelin and desacyl ghrelin concentrations in renal failure. J Am Soc Nephrol 2002;13:2748–2752.
62 Aygen B, Dogukan A, Dursun FE, Aydin S, Kilic N, et al: Ghrelin and obestatin levels in end-stage renal disease. J Int Med Res 2009;37:757–765.
63 Lainscak M, Andreas S, Scanlon PD, Somers VK, Anker SD: Ghrelin and neurohumoral antagonists in the treatment of cachexia associated with cardiopulmonary disease. Intern Med 2006;45:837.
64 Itoh T, Nagaya N, Yoshikawa M, Fukuoka A, Takenaka H, et al: Elevated plasma ghrelin level in underweight patients with chronic obstructive pulmonary disease. Am J Respir Crit Care Med 2004;170:879–882.
65 Shimizu Y, Nagaya N, Isobe T, Imazu M, Okumura H, et al: Increased plasma ghrelin level in lung cancer cachexia. Clin Cancer Res 2003;9:774–778.
66 Garcia JM, Garcia-Touza M, Hijazi RA, Taffet G, Epner D, et al: Active ghrelin levels and active to total ghrelin ratio in cancer-induced cachexia. J Clin Endocrinol Metab 2005;90:2920–2926.
67 Wolf I, Sadetzki S, Kanety H, Kundel Y, Pariente C, et al: Adiponectin, ghrelin, and leptin in cancer cachexia in breast and colon cancer patients. Cancer 2006;106:966–973.
68 Williams DL, Cummings DE: Regulation of ghrelin in physiologic and pathophysiologic states. J Nutr 2005;135:1320–1325.
69 Kirchner H, Gutierrez JA, Solenberg PJ, Pfluger PT, Czyzyk TA, et al: GOAT links dietary lipids with the endocrine control of energy balance. Nat Med 2009;15:741–745.

70 Perez-Tilve D, Heppner K, Kirchner H, Lockie SH, Woods SC, et al: Ghrelin-induced adiposity is independent of orexigenic effects. FASEB J 2011;25: 2814–2822.
71 Barsh GS, Schwartz MW: Genetic approaches to studying energy balance: perception and integration. Nat Rev Genet 2002;3:589–600.
72 Kamegai J, Tamura H, Shimizu T, Ishii S, Sugihara H, et al: Central effect of ghrelin, an endogenous growth hormone secretagogue, on hypothalamic peptide gene expression. Endocrinology 2000;141: 4797–4800.
73 Kamegai J, Tamura H, Shimizu T, Ishii S, Sugihara H, et al: Chronic central infusion of ghrelin increases hypothalamic neuropeptide Y and Agouti-related protein mRNA levels and body weight in rats. Diabetes 2001;50:2438–2443.
74 Nakazato M, Murakami N, Date Y, Kojima M, Matsuo H, et al: A role for ghrelin in the central regulation of feeding. Nature 2001;409:194–198.
75 Theander-Carrillo C, Wiedmer P, Cettour-Rose P, Nogueiras R, Perez-Tilve D, et al: Ghrelin action in the brain controls adipocyte metabolism. J Clin Invest 2006;116:1983–1993.
76 von Haehling S, Lainscak M, Springer J, Anker SD: Cardiac cachexia: a systematic overview. Pharmacol Ther 2009;121:227–252.
77 Ashby D, Choi P, Bloom S: Gut hormones and the treatment of disease cachexia. Proc Nutr Soc 2008; 67:263–269.
78 Muller TD, Perez-Tilve D, Tong J, Pfluger PT, Tschop MH: Ghrelin and its potential in the treatment of eating/wasting disorders and cachexia. J Cachexia Sarcopenia Muscle 2010;1:159–167.
79 Ashitani J, Matsumoto N, Nakazato M: Ghrelin and its therapeutic potential for cachectic patients. Peptides 2009;30:1951–1956.
80 Langhans W: Peripheral mechanisms involved with catabolism. Curr Opin Clin Nutr Metab Care 2002; 5:419–426.
81 Hebebrand J, Muller TD, Holtkamp K, Herpertz-Dahlmann B. The role of leptin in anorexia nervosa: clinical implications. Mol Psychiatry 2007;12:23–35.
82 Otto B, Cuntz U, Fruehauf E, Wawarta R, Folwaczny C, et al: Weight gain decreases elevated plasma ghrelin concentrations of patients with anorexia nervosa. Eur J Endocrinol 2001;145:669–673.
83 Otto B, Tschop M, Fruhauf E, Heldwein W, Fichter M, et al: Postprandial ghrelin release in anorectic patients before and after weight gain. Psychoneuroendocrinology 2005;30:577–581.
84 Haas V, Onur S, Paul T, Nutzinger DO, Bosy-Westphal A, et al: Leptin and body weight regulation in patients with anorexia nervosa before and during weight recovery. Am J Clin Nutr 2005;81:889–896.
85 Germain N, Galusca B, Grouselle D, Frere D, Tolle V, et al: Ghrelin/obestatin ratio in two populations with low bodyweight: constitutional thinness and anorexia nervosa. Psychoneuroendocrinology 2009; 34:413–419.
86 Druce MR, Wren AM, Park AJ, Milton JE, Patterson M, et al: Ghrelin increases food intake in obese as well as lean subjects. Int J Obes (Lond) 2009;29: 1130–1136.
87 Wren AM, Seal LJ, Cohen MA, Brynes AE, Frost GS, et al: Ghrelin enhances appetite and increases food intake in humans. J Clin Endocrinol Metab 2001;86: 5992.
88 Garcia JM, Polvino WJ: Effect on body weight and safety of RC-1291, a novel, orally available ghrelin mimetic and growth hormone secretagogue: results of a phase I, randomized, placebo-controlled, multiple-dose study in healthy volunteers. Oncologist 2007;12:594–600.
89 Hotta M, Ohwada R, Akamizu T, Shibasaki T, Takano K, et al: Ghrelin increases hunger and food intake in patients with restricting-type anorexia nervosa: a pilot study. Endocr J 2009;56:1119–1128.
90 Burdet L, de Muralt B, Schutz Y, Pichard C, Fitting JW: Administration of growth hormone to underweight patients with chronic obstructive pulmonary disease. A prospective, randomized, controlled study. Am J Respir Crit Care Med 1997;156:1800–1806.
91 Nagaya N, Kangawa K: Ghrelin, a novel growth hormone-releasing peptide, in the treatment of chronic heart failure. Regul Pept 2003;114:71–77.
92 Nagaya N, Kangawa K: Ghrelin improves left ventricular dysfunction and cardiac cachexia in heart failure. Curr Opin Pharmacol 2003;3:146–151.
93 Nagaya N, Uematsu M, Kojima M, Ikeda Y, Yoshihara F, et al: Chronic administration of ghrelin improves left ventricular dysfunction and attenuates development of cardiac cachexia in rats with heart failure. Circulation 2001;104:1430–1435.
94 Xu XB, Pang JJ, Cao JM, Ni C, Xu RK, et al: GH-releasing peptides improve cardiac dysfunction and cachexia and suppress stress-related hormones and cardiomyocyte apoptosis in rats with heart failure. Am J Physiol Heart Circ Physiol 2005;289:H1643–H1651.
95 Deboer MD, Zhu X, Levasseur PR, Inui A, Hu Z, et al: Ghrelin treatment of chronic kidney disease: improvements in lean body mass and cytokine profile. Endocrinology 2008;149:827–835.
96 Hanada T, Toshinai K, Kajimura N, Nara-Ashizawa N, Tsukada T, et al: Anti-cachectic effect of ghrelin in nude mice bearing human melanoma cells. Biochem Biophys Res Commun 2003;301:275–279.

97 Hanada T, Toshinai K, Date Y, Kajimura N, Tsukada T, et al: Upregulation of ghrelin expression in cachectic nude mice bearing human melanoma cells. Metabolism 2004;53:84–88.
98 DeBoer MD, Zhu XX, Levasseur P, Meguid MM, Suzuki S, et al: Ghrelin treatment causes increased food intake and retention of lean body mass in a rat model of cancer cachexia. Endocrinology 2007;148: 3004–3012.
99 Wynne K, Giannitsopoulou K, Small CJ, Patterson M, Frost G, et al: Subcutaneous ghrelin enhances acute food intake in malnourished patients who receive maintenance peritoneal dialysis: a randomized, placebo-controlled trial. J Am Soc Nephrol 2005;16:2111–2118.
100 Ashby DR, Ford HE, Wynne KJ, Wren AM, Murphy KG, et al: Sustained appetite improvement in malnourished dialysis patients by daily ghrelin treatment. Kidney Int 2009;76:199–206.
101 Nagaya N, Moriya J, Yasumura Y, Uematsu M, Ono F, et al: Effects of ghrelin administration on left ventricular function, exercise capacity, and muscle wasting in patients with chronic heart failure. Circulation 2004;110:3674–3679.
102 Nagaya N, Itoh T, Murakami S, Oya H, Uematsu M, et al: Treatment of cachexia with ghrelin in patients with COPD. Chest 2005;128:1187–1193.
103 Neary NM, Small CJ, Wren AM, Lee JL, Druce MR, et al: Ghrelin increases energy intake in cancer patients with impaired appetite: acute, randomized, placebo-controlled trial. J Clin Endocrinol Metab 2004;89:2832–2836.
104 Strasser F, Lutz TA, Maeder MT, Thuerlimann B, Bueche D, et al: Safety, tolerability and pharmacokinetics of intravenous ghrelin for cancer-related anorexia/cachexia: a randomised, placebo-controlled, double-blind, double-crossover study. Br J Cancer 2008;98:300–308.

Prof. Matthias H. Tschöp
Institute for Diabetes and Obesity, Helmholtz Zentrum München and Department of Medicine
Technische Universität München
DE–85764 Munich (Germany)
E-Mail tschoep@helmholtz-muenchen.de

Benso A, Casanueva FF, Ghigo E, Granata A (eds): The Ghrelin System.
Endocr Dev. Basel, Karger, 2013, vol 25, pp 101–111 (DOI: 10.1159/000346058)

Ghrelin, Reward and Motivation

John R.W. Menzies[a] · Karolina P. Skibicka[b] · Gareth Leng[a] · Suzanne L. Dickson[b]

[a]Centre for Integrative Physiology, School of Biomedical Sciences, University of Edinburgh, Edinburgh, UK; [b]Department of Physiology/Endocrinology, Institute of Neuroscience and Physiology, The Sahlgrenska Academy at the University of Gothenburg, Gothenburg, Sweden

Abstract
Almost all circulating gut peptides contribute to the control of food intake by signalling satiety. One important exception is ghrelin, the only orexigenic peptide hormone thus far described. Ghrelin secretion increases before meals and behavioural and electrophysiological evidence shows that ghrelin acts in the hypothalamus via homeostatic pathways to signal hunger and increase food intake and adiposity. These findings strongly suggest that ghrelin is a dynamically regulated peripheral hunger signal. However, ghrelin also interacts with the brain reward pathways to increase food intake, alter food preference and enhance food reward. Here we discuss ghrelin's role as an endocrine gut-brain reward signal in relation to homeostatic and hedonic feeding control.

We are bombarded fairly steadily by reports of a high and rising incidence of obesity. Being obese is not in itself a problem but the consequences of obesity, like type 2 diabetes, cardiovascular diseases and some cancers, are of concern. Food intake is controlled by the brain but what, how much and how often we eat is not only driven by homeostatic requirements for calories and nutrients. The existence of what is now labelled an obesity epidemic is evidence that many people must have a strong drive to eat even when homeostatic signals indicate a positive energy balance in the form of large fat stores. However, we do not eat only for energy and nutrients, we also eat for pleasure. The target for hedonic-driven eating is a broad category of palatable foods with certain characteristics in common. Unfortunately, the foods we enjoy the most tend not to be nutritionally balanced, but are high in sugar, fat, salt and calories. What is more, hedonic desire for palatable foods can easily inundate the homeostatic mechanisms that normally delay the start or signal the termination of feeding. Thus, reward-driven feeding may drive and support overeating, weight gain, obesity and illness.

How might this happen? There are several possibilities – firstly, changes in the reward system may be a secondary effect of the onset or maintenance of obesity. The central signal most strongly associated with the reinforcing effects of palatable food is dopamine released from the mesolimbic structures. In humans, striatal dopamine receptor number is reduced in obesity [1] and this may be linked to a blunting of the normal reward response to food. When neural activity in the striatum is monitored in response to palatable food ingestion, individuals show reduced reward responses to an identical stimulus after having gained weight [2]. Secondly, and perhaps in contrast to this neuroadaptive reprogramming theory, a pre-existing genetic or epigenetic susceptibility or sensitivity to reward may exist. For example, striatal D2 receptor expression shows interindividual differences related to body weight. But rather than an obesity-driven mechanism, inherent differences in expression of the A1 allele of the TaqIA polymorphism may underlie this [3]. Selectively bred lines of obesity-prone rats (whose phenotypes presumably reflect subtle genetic differences from obesity-resistant rats) show several impairments in proteins involved in dopamine neurotransmission. These are evident before exposure to a palatable diet or excess weight gain [4]. Thirdly, the consumption of palatable food may be considered to be a form of addiction. In experiments loosely parallel to those of Olds [5] where rats crossed electrified grids to self-stimulate their brain reward centres, rats made obese by chronic access to palatable food will continue to eat such food even when conditioned to associate its consumption with a painful electric shock [6]. In other words, reward-related stimuli may compel the consumption of palatable food even in the face of marked negative outcomes, real or potential – a classical attribute of addiction [7]. None of these three possibilities are mutually-exclusive and other aspects of the reward system may also be important. It is not yet clear whether reward-related obesity may be a consequence of hyper- or hypoactivity of the reward system. However, there may be strong parallels with other addictive disorders. Hyperactivity of the reward system likely drives initial overconsumption of rewarding food but then the behaviour becomes reinforced and habitual rather than enjoyable. A hedonic deficit may develop which is compensated for by increased motivation or a craving for the rewarding food. This may result in sustained 'wanting' in the absence of 'liking'. In other words, eating *without* pleasure.

In any case, the power of the reward system over feeding behaviour should not be underestimated. Compared with homeostatic mechanisms of feeding, much less is currently known about how hedonic systems in the brain influence food intake. It is clear, however, that hormonal peptide signals converge on certain brain regions and are pivotal in both homeostatic and hedonic feeding. Ghrelin is a naturally occurring peptide that is found in several regions of the body, including the brain, but is predominantly synthesised in the mucosal cells of the stomach. Ghrelin is secreted into the blood, levels rise during periods of energy depletion, including between normally-spaced meals, and fall upon feeding. Ghrelin acts centrally to signal hunger and, via well-characterised hypothalamic pathways, increases food intake in humans and rodents [8]. In addition, accumulating evidence points to a role for ghrelin in the modulation of motivation and reward, not only in feeding but also in responses to artificial rewards such as alcohol. Here, we review the target reward pathways for ghrelin, the receptors and neurobiological substrates of importance for ghrelin's effects on food intake, food reward and food motivated behaviour.

Ghrelin's Influence on Central Reward Pathways

The central reward pathways comprise multiple interconnected brain regions many of which are sensitive to hormonal peptides commonly associated with the control of homeostatic feeding [9]. The best-characterised pathway (now approaching 'classical' status) is the dopaminergic innervation of the nucleus accumbens (NAcc) by neurones in the ventral tegmental area (VTA). Other regions, especially the target sites of the NAcc such as the prefrontal cortex and ventral pallidum, and inputs into the NAcc such as the amygdala, are also important for reward processing. Other regions implicated in ghrelin signalling such as the lateral and ventromedial hypothalamus and the arcuate nucleus also form neurocircuits with the reward pathways that are likely to be important in integrating feeding control [10]. The ghrelin (GHS-R1A) receptor is localised in many brain regions associated with pleasure, reward and motivation. An early report noted GHS-R1A receptor mRNA expression in the substantia nigra and VTA and speculated whether receptor localisation in the reward pathway may indicate a role for the then-unidentified endogenous ligand in hedonic motivation [11]. Further evidence comes from studies using biotin-labelled ghrelin which binds to VTA neurones with a similar pattern of distribution seen to GHS-R1A receptor immunoreactivity [12]. GHS-R1A mRNA is translated to express functional ghrelin receptors in VTA neurones and ghrelin administration to this region causes dopamine release [12, 13], although this may be dependent on feeding state [14]. Ghrelin excites VTA neurones in brain slices in vitro [12] and increases dopamine activity (as measured by the DOPAC:dopamine ratio or by microdialysis to directly measure dopamine release in the NAcc) in wild-type and ghrelin knockout mice but not in GHS-R1A receptor knockout mice [12, 13, 15].

Ghrelin and Natural Rewards: Food and Sex

Readers of this book hardly need to be reminded of ghrelin's central role in food intake. However, the discovery of the peptide solved an apparent mystery. Initially, the presence of GHS-R1A receptors in brain regions associated with food intake was not easily explained, particularly as most interested parties considered this receptor to be the target for a class of synthetic growth hormone secretagogues and, as such, are presumably mainly involved in the control of growth hormone secretion by an endoge-

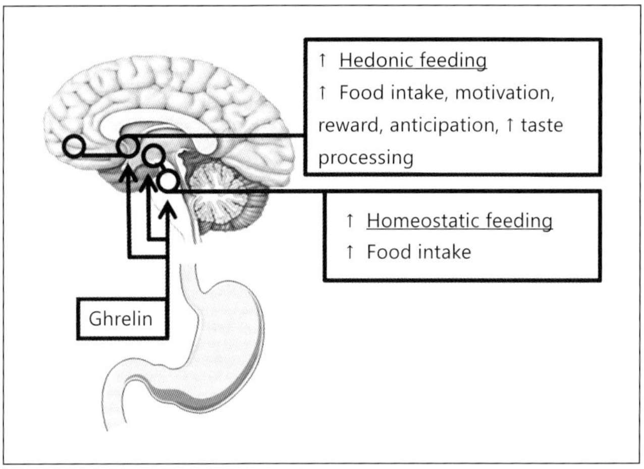

Fig. 1. A simplified illustration of brain regions sensitive to ghrelin. Ghrelin is secreted from the stomach into the blood to activate at least two distinct brain pathways involved in feeding. Activation of the homeostatic hypothalamus drives food intake. In addition to food intake, activation of hedonic pathways can also affect motivation and anticipation for food.

nous ligand. Aware of the localisation of somatostatin- and GHRH-containing neurones for example, most expected a hypothalamic source for an endogenous GHS-R1A ligand, perhaps released from neuroendocrine cells into the blood to target somatotrophs. The finding that ghrelin was synthesised in and secreted from the stomach was unanticipated, even by its discoverers [16, 17]. The peptide's localisation in the stomach and the localisation of GHS-R1A receptors in the arcuate and ventromedial nuclei drove a clear research direction addressing potential roles in food intake. Very soon ghrelin was shown to have effects on food intake, body weight and body composition in rodents [18–20] and evidence for changes in obese or anorexic humans followed [21, 22]. Several years' productive effort was focused on ghrelin's role in the homeostatic control of feeding, mainly via its direct excitatory action at orexigenic NPY/AgRP/GABA neurones in the hypothalamic arcuate and ventromedial nuclei. Latterly though, attention has turned to the reward pathway as an important target [9, 23].

Ghrelin induces an acute orexigenic response when administered peripherally [24] or directly into the brain ventricles [25]. In 2005, Naleid et al. [27] demonstrated an orexigenic response following direct administration of low doses of ghrelin into the VTA and also the NAcc [26], a finding that we have since been able to replicate. This was the first indication that ghrelin may provide a gut-brain reward signal that is linked to feeding control at the level of the reward system. It seems rather likely that ghrelin accesses these reward circuits, especially as peripheral ghrelin injection has been shown to increase accumbal dopamine release [13]. The afferent stimulus provided by ghrelin could also be derived centrally, although it remains much debated whether ghrelin is produced in the brain as many research groups, including our own, have been unable to detect ghrelin mRNA in the brain by in situ hybridization. It can also be questioned whether an afferent ghrelin signal is required for GHS-R1A activation as the receptor appears to have constitutive activity in the absence of ligand [28]

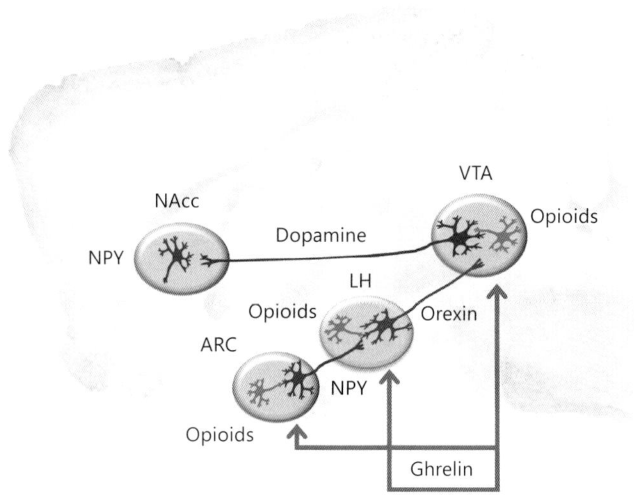

Fig. 2. Schematic illustration of brain pathways mediating ghrelin's effects on food motivation. A key pathway involved in food motivation is the midbrain dopamine projection from the VTA to the NAcc. Ghrelin appears to activate this pathway directly at the level of the VTA. This provides a potential mechanism for ghrelin to promote food intake even when homeostatic hypothalamic centres such as the arcuate nucleus (ARC) or lateral hypothalamus (LH) indicate a state of satiety. It is also possible that ghrelin affects food motivation indirectly, for example, by activating an afferent pathway. Recent studies suggest that while central opioid (via the mu receptor) and NPY (Y1 receptor) signalling are required for ghrelin's effects on food motivation, the targets sites for these effects differ. At the level of the VTA, opioid signalling (but not NPY signalling) is required for ghrelin's effects on food motivation [39].

and may be able to modify dopamine signalling by heterodimerising with dopamine D1 receptors in, for example, ghrelin-sensitive neurones in the VTA [29].

The basic goal of feeding is to acquire calories and a diversity of nutrients. There is an obvious advantage in being able to detect a food high in energy, and one excellent indicator of this nutritional property is sweetness. Mammals appear to have an innate pre-disposition to preferentially eat sweet foods. Remarkably, rats trained to make a mutually exclusive choice between a behaviourally effective i.v. dose of cocaine or a short period of access to a sweet drink show a strong and sustained preference for the sweet taste [30]. Evidence suggests that ghrelin signalling may play an essential role in the motivation to consume sweet food over bland food. When given a free choice between bland food or sweet, palatable, energy-dense food, GHS-R1A receptor knockout mice and mice treated with a GHS-R1A receptor antagonist eat less palatable food than controls. Furthermore, palatable food consumption is usually associated with an increase in dopamine release in the NAcc but this is not observed in GHS-R1A knockouts [31]. In mice, the ability of sweet chocolate treats to condition a place preference is abolished by peripheral treatment with a GHS-R1A receptor antagonist [31] and is absent in fasted GHS-R1A receptor knockout mice [32]. Access to a pelleted high-fat rodent diet also conditions a place preference in mice. This is enhanced by ghrelin administered peripherally but GHS-R1A receptor knockout mice show no such preference [33].

Building on serendipitous findings by Constantin Fahlberg in 1878, chemists are now able to produce molecules that are many hundred times sweeter than sucrose. These can therefore be used at very low concentrations, low enough to provide next to non-metabolisable energy. Saccharin is the prototypical artificial sweetener and rats will preferentially consume sweet-tasting saccharin solutions over water [34] but not in preference to approximately equally sweet natural, calorific sugars [35]. This gives rise to the idea of at least two aspects of reward driven by differing qualities in different foods; a gustatory reward (the pleasure of taste) and a post-ingestive reward (the pleasure associated with changes in plasma nutrient or hormonal levels). In addition to increasing sweet, caloric food intake, ghrelin also enhances sweet, non-caloric saccharin intake both in the presence and absence of caloric food. Also, consumption of a saccharin-sweetened food is reduced in GHS-R1A knockout mice compared to wild-type mice [36].

If an animal finds food rewarding, it will show motivated behaviour to obtain it. This can be demonstrated in an operant conditioning paradigm in which rats must work progressively harder in order to obtain a sweet treat. Motivated behaviour for a sucrose reward is increased by ghrelin given centrally or peripherally to satiated rats and, conversely, is suppressed in hungry rats by a GHS-R1A antagonist, also administered by these routes [37]. Indeed ghrelin administration directly to the VTA, but not the NAcc, increases food-motivated behaviour, thereby identifying the VTA as the primary target for these effects of ghrelin [37]. Consistent with this, chemical lesion of the VTA reduces ghrelin-evoked food-motivated behaviour [38]. Using the same operant self-administration model of motivation for sucrose, pharmacological blockade of NPY receptors with intracentroventricular administration of a selective Y1 receptor antagonist prevents a ghrelin-evoked increase in motivation. This observation is recapitulated with an opioid receptor antagonist. In contrast, ghrelin's local effects in the VTA on intake of normal bland food are unaffected by opioid receptor antagonism but are reduced by Y1 receptor blockade [39]. Interestingly, intra-VTA infusion of NPY antagonist does not prevent the potentiating effect of ghrelin on motivation suggesting that NPY activation to increase food motivation is at an extra-VTA site, possibly the lateral hypothalamus or NAcc [39]. Taken together, this indicates that central NPY and opioid receptor activation is required for ghrelin's enhancement of sucrose motivation, but that in the VTA only opioid receptors are utilised by ghrelin for this response.

An important aspect of feeding-related behaviour is locomotion. An animal must forage or hunt for food before it can eat it. Ghrelin increases locomotion in mice when given centrally into the third ventricle [15] or more locally in the VTA or LDTg [13, 31]. Rats fed for a restricted period each day quickly develop food-entrained anticipatory activity (FAA) where a marked increase in locomotion is seen several hours prior to the time food is expected. Plasma ghrelin levels are specifically increased during a conditioned period of FAA in rats and physical activity levels can be reduced by intracebrovascular injection of a GHS-R1A receptor antagonist prior to the expected FAA [40]. Furthermore, decreased levels of FAA are observed in GHS-R1A receptor knockout mice. As well as conditioning FAA by restricted access to normal food, FAA can be evoked by restricted presentation of a palatable food in addition to ad lib access to normal food. When rats are given restricted access to a small amount of chocolate they show FAA similar to that seen in food-restricted animals and plasma ghrelin levels are elevated compared to rats not anticipating the palatable reward. In addition, intracebrovascular ghrelin increases FAA for a reward while intracebrovascular administration of a GHS-R1A receptor antagonist decreases it [41]. Thus, ghrelin appears to have a role in anticipatory activity for food, both predicted meals when hungry and predicted additional food rewards when satiated.

What cellular and molecular mechanisms might underlie this important role for ghrelin in reward and motivation? After chronic intracebrovascular ghrelin administration in rats, VTA dopamine D5 receptor mRNA and nicotinic acetylcholine nAChRb2 receptor mRNA expression are increased whereas in the NAcc, there is reduced mRNA expression of dopamine D1A, D3 and D5 receptors and reduced expression of nicotinic acetylcholine nAChRa3 receptors [37]. Acute ghrelin administration to the VTA also upregulates opioid receptor mRNA in VTA neurones [39]. While it remains to be determined whether these molecular-level changes are simply compensatory responses to an enhanced dopamine signal for example, it is possible they could directly contribute to the rewarding effects of ghrelin. An increase in opioid receptor expression may underlie the interaction between ghrelin and opioids in the VTA, where a reward stimulus can elicit opioid release and concurrent ghrelin sensitises the VTA neuronal response to opioids by increasing opioid receptor expression. The presence of ghrelin could, therefore, make the stimulus of a single food reward much more motivating.

Less evidence exists for a role for ghrelin in modifying food reward in humans. Experiments measuring hunger or the wanting and liking of foods in human subjects can be contentious, relying as they often do on subjective experience or self-reporting. However, in an fMRI study using satiated human subjects exposed to images of palatable foods, ghrelin increased a BOLD response in likely neural correlates of reward pathway activation such as the amygdala, orbitofrontal cortex and anterior insula, but not in the homeostatic hypothalamus [42].

Animals perform many natural goal-oriented behaviours that result in pleasure and reinforcement. After eating and drinking, the next most common of these is sexual behaviour. Ghrelin has a partially characterised effect on hormonal reproductive physiology via actions on the hypothalamo-pituitary-gonadal axis. Ghrelin, like leptin, may be involved in the metabolic gating of the onset of puberty. For example, high plasma ghrelin levels may signal that insufficient energy is available for the demands of sexual maturation [43]. In contrast, much less is known about a potential role for ghrelin in sexual motivation and reward. In male mice administered an orexigenic dose of ghrelin, ultrasonic calling (a pre-copulatory courting behaviour) is reduced but the strong preference for females' bedding observed in controls is neither enhanced nor reduced by ghrelin administration [44]. For males, sexual behaviour is not particularly costly, so moderate hunger (reflected by levels of ghrelin high in the physiological range) may not be a sufficient obstacle to prevent males taking advantage of an opportunity to mate [45]. Nonetheless, it may be of interest to carefully determine the effects of ghrelin on a place preference conditioned by a receptive female or her odour, on sexual incentive motivation tests or on the latency or number of intromissions when male animals are allowed access to receptive females. In contrast to males, reproduction for females is extremely energetically expensive. In the context of reproduction perhaps energy stores are of more significance in females and sexual behaviours may be more susceptible to modification by energy balance signals. Indeed, fasting or acute but not chronic ghrelin treatment can reduce sexual receptivity in female rats [46].

Conclusion: Ghrelin as a Reward Amplifier?

From an evolutionary perspective, ghrelin signalling may provide a strong driving force to ensure both an adequate nutritional supply and a diversity of food of varying reward value. It makes physiological sense that the empty stomach signals to neurocircuits involved in food motivation and craving, but this system can be hijacked by obesogenic foods in the modern Western lifestyle, contributing strongly to the development of obesity. What is more, the effects of ghrelin on reward are not confined to natural rewards. Suppressed ghrelin signalling interrupts reward from chemical drugs of abuse such as alcohol [47], nicotine [48], cocaine and amphetamine [49]. Moreover, central ghrelin injection increases drug consumption and behaviours associated with the motivation for drugs. It should be noted, however, that ghrelin administration is itself rewarding, mice will show preference for an environment previously paired with ghrelin administration [50].

Possible targets for treatment by drugs modifying central ghrelin signalling are obesity, hypophagic diseases such as anorexia and forms of drug and alcohol abuse. The most prevalent of these is of course obesity. It is worthwhile noting that changes in circulating ghrelin are seen in obesity and after its treatment by bariatric surgery [51]. Furthermore, the concept of ghrelin resistance in homeostatic neural circuits after diet-induced obesity has been suggested [52], paralleling that of leptin resistance and insulin resistance manifesting as type 2 diabetes. Extending this idea to the motivation to eat, mice made obese by a high-fat diet are less motivated to obtain food rewards in basal conditions and after ghrelin treatment; diet-induced obesity suppresses the stimulatory effect of ghrelin compared to lean mice [53]. It can be argued whether a major physiological role of ghrelin is to drive hunger or prevent starvation but it is certain that ghrelin is orexigenic. Ghrelin's actions in food motivation complement this pro-feeding effect. It is clear that ghrelin is an important gut-brain signal for food intake driven by energy deficit or by an anticipated reward value.

Acknowledgements

Supported by the European Community's Seventh Framework Programme (FP7/2007–2013) under grant agreements No. 245009 (NeuroFAST, www.neurofast.eu), No. 266408 (Full4Health, www.full4health.eu) and n°241592 (EurOCHIP, www.eurochip-obesity.com), the Swedish Research Council for Medicine (2011–3054 to K.P.S., 2009-S266 to S.L.D., 12208, 2009–2618), FOU/ALF Göteborg (ALFGBG-138741), NovoNordisk Fonden and the Swedish Foundation for Strategic Research to Sahlgrenska Center for Cardiovascular and Metabolic Research (A305–188) 5–4328.

References

1 Volkow ND, Wang GJ, Telang F, Fowler JS, Thanos PK, Logan J, Alexoff D, Ding YS, Wong C, Ma Y, Pradhan K: Low dopamine striatal D2 receptors are associated with prefrontal metabolism in obese subjects: possible contributing factors. Neuroimage 2008;42:1537–1543.

2 Stice E, Yokum S, Blum K, Bohon C: Weight gain is associated with reduced striatal response to palatable food. J Neurosci 2010;30:13105–13109.

3 Stice E, Spoor S, Bohon C, Small DM: Relation between obesity and blunted striatal response to food is moderated by TaqIA A1 allele. Science 2008;322:449–452.

4 Geiger BM, Behr GG, Frank LE, Caldera-Siu AD, Beinfeld MC, Kokkotou EG, Pothos EN: Evidence for defective mesolimbic dopamine exocytosis in obesity-prone rats. FASEB J 2008;22:2740–2746.

5 Olds J: Self-stimulation of the brain: its use to study local effects of hunger, sex, and drugs. Science 1958;127:315–324.

6 Johnson PM, Kenny PJ: Dopamine D2 receptors in addiction-like reward dysfunction and compulsive eating in obese rats. Nat Neurosci 2010;13:635–641.

7 Avena NM, Rada P, Hoebel BG: Evidence for sugar addiction: behavioral and neurochemical effects of intermittent, excessive sugar intake. Neurosci Biobehav Rev 2008;32:20–39.

8 van der Lely AJ, Tschöp M, Heiman ML, Ghigo E: Biological, physiological, pathophysiological, and pharmacological aspects of ghrelin. Endocr Rev 2004;25:426–457.

9 Menzies JRW, Skibicka KP, Egecioglu E, Leng G, Dickson SL: Peripheral signals modifying food reward. Handb Exp Pharmacol 2012;209:131–158.

10 Scott V, McDade DM, Luckman SM: Rapid changes in the sensitivity of arcuate nucleus neurons to central ghrelin in relation to feeding status. Physiol Behav 2007;90:180–185.

11 Guan XM, Yu H, Palyha OC, McKee KK, Feighner SD, Sirinathsinghji DJ, Smith RG, Van der Ploeg LH, Howard AD: Distribution of mRNA encoding the growth hormone secretagogue receptor in brain and peripheral tissues. Brain Res Mol Brain Res 1997;48:23–29.

12 Abizaid A, Liu ZW, Andrews ZB, Shanabrough M, Borok E, Elsworth JD, Roth RH, Sleeman MW, Picciotto MR, Tschöp MH, Gao XB, Horvath TL: Ghrelin modulates the activity and synaptic input organization of midbrain dopamine neurons while promoting appetite. J Clin Invest 2006;116:3229–3239.

13 Jerlhag E, Egecioglu E, Dickson SL, Douhan A, Svensson L, Engel JA: Ghrelin administration into tegmental areas stimulates locomotor activity and increases extracellular concentration of dopamine in the nucleus accumbens. Addict Biol 2007;12:6–16.

14 Kawahara Y, Kawahara H, Kaneko F, Yamada M, Nishi Y, Tanaka E, Nishi A: Peripherally administered ghrelin induces bimodal effects on the mesolimbic dopamine system depending on food-consumptive states. Neuroscience 2009;161:855–864.

15 Jerlhag E, Egecioglu E, Dickson SL, Andersson M, Svensson L, Engel JA: Ghrelin stimulates locomotor activity and accumbal dopamine-overflow via central cholinergic systems in mice: implications for its involvement in brain reward. Addict Biol 2006;11:45–54.

16 Kojima M, Hosoda H, Date Y, Nakazato M, Matsuo H, Kangawa K: Ghrelin is a growth-hormone-releasing acylated peptide from stomach. Nature 1999;402: 656–660.
17 Kojima M: The discovery of ghrelin – a personal memory. Regul Pept 2008;145:2–6.
18 Tschöp M, Smiley DL, Heiman ML: Ghrelin induces adiposity in rodents. Nature 2000;407:908–913.
19 Wren AM, Small CJ, Ward HL, Murphy KG, Dakin CL, Taheri S, Kennedy AR, Roberts GH, Morgan DG, Ghatei MA, Bloom SR: The novel hypothalamic peptide ghrelin stimulates food intake and growth hormone secretion. Endocrinology 2000;141:4325–4328.
20 Nakazato M, Murakami N, Date Y, Kojima M, Matsuo H, Kangawa K, Matsukura S: A role for ghrelin in the central regulation of feeding. Nature 2001;409: 194–198.
21 Otto B, Cuntz U, Fruehauf E, Wawarta R, Folwaczny C, Riepl RL, Heiman ML, Lehnert P, Fichter M, Tschöp M: Weight gain decreases elevated plasma ghrelin concentrations of patients with anorexia nervosa. Eur J Endocrinol 2001;145:669–673.
22 Tschöp M, Weyer C, Tataranni PA, Devanarayan V, Ravussin E, Heiman ML: Circulating ghrelin levels are decreased in human obesity. Diabetes 2001;50: 707–709.
23 Skibicka KP, Dickson SL: Ghrelin and food reward: the story of potential underlying substrates. Peptides 2011;32:2265–2273.
24 Wren AM, Small CJ, Abbott CR, Dhillo WS, Seal LJ, Cohen MA, Batterham RL, Taheri S, Stanley SA, Ghatei MA, Bloom SR: Ghrelin causes hyperphagia and obesity in rats. Diabetes 2001;50:2540–2547.
25 Asakawa A, Inui A, Kaga T, Yuzuriha H, Nagata T, Ueno N, Makino S, Fujimiya M, Niijima A, Fujino MA, Kasuga M: Ghrelin is an appetite-stimulatory signal from stomach with structural resemblance to motilin. Gastroenterology 2001;120:337–345.
26 Naleid AM, Grace MK, Cummings DE, Levine AS: Ghrelin induces feeding in the mesolimbic reward pathway between the ventral tegmental area and the nucleus accumbens. Peptides 2005;26:2274–2279.
27 Skibicka KP, Hansson C, Alvarez-Crespo M, Friberg PA, Dickson SL: Ghrelin directly targets the ventral tegmental area to increase food motivation. Neuroscience 2011;180:129–137.
28 Holst B, Cygankiewicz A, Jensen TH, Ankersen M, Schwartz TW: High constitutive signaling of the ghrelin receptor – identification of a potent inverse agonist. Mol Endocrinol 2003;17:2201–2210.
29 Jiang H, Betancourt L, Smith RG: Ghrelin amplifies dopamine signaling by cross talk involving formation of growth hormone secretagogue receptor/dopamine receptor subtype 1 heterodimers. Mol Endocrinol 2006;20:1772–1785.
30 Lenoir M, Serre F, Cantin L, Ahmed SH: Intense sweetness surpasses cocaine reward. PLoS One 2007; 2:e698.
31 Egecioglu E, Jerlhag E, Salomé N, Skibicka KP, Haage D, Bohlooly-Y M, Andersson D, Bjursell M, Perrissoud D, Engel JA, Dickson SL: Ghrelin increases intake of rewarding food in rodents. Addict Biol 2010;15:304–311.
32 Disse E, Bussier AL, Deblon N, Pfluger PT, Tschöp MH, Laville M, Rohner-Jeanrenaud F: Systemic ghrelin and reward: effect of cholinergic blockade. Physiol Behav 2011;102:481–484.
33 Perello M, Sakata I, Birnbaum S, Chuang JC, Osborne-Lawrence S, Rovinsky SA, Woloszyn J, Yanagisawa M, Lutter M, Zigman JM: Ghrelin increases the rewarding value of high-fat diet in an orexin-dependent manner. Biol Psychiatry 2010;67:880–886.
34 Tordoff MG, Alarcon LK, Lawler MP: Preferences of 14 rat strains for 17 taste compounds. Physiol Behav 2008;95:308–332.
35 Domingos AI, Vaynshteyn J, Voss HU, Ren X, Gradinaru V, Zang F, Deisseroth K, de Araujo IE, Friedman J: Leptin regulates the reward value of nutrient. Nat Neurosci 2011;14:1562–1568.
36 Disse E, Bussier AL, Veyrat-Durebex C, Deblon N, Pfluger PT, Tschöp MH, Laville M, Rohner-Jeanrenaud F: Peripheral ghrelin enhances sweet taste food consumption and preference, regardless of its caloric content. Physiol Behav 2010;101:277–281.
37 Skibicka KP, Hansson C, Egecioglu E, Dickson SL: Role of ghrelin in food reward: impact of ghrelin on sucrose self-administration and mesolimbic dopamine and acetylcholine receptor gene expression. Addict Biol 2012;17:95–107.
38 Weinberg ZY, Nicholson ML, Currie PJ: 6-Hydroxydopamine lesions of the ventral tegmental area suppress ghrelin's ability to elicit food-reinforced behavior. Neurosci Lett 2011;499:70–73.
39 Skibicka KP, Shirazi RH, Hansson C, Dickson SL: Ghrelin interacts with neuropeptide Y Y1 and opioid receptors to increase food reward. Endocrinology 2012;153:1194–1205.
40 Verhagen LA, Egecioglu E, Luijendijk MC, Hillebrand JJ, Adan RA, Dickson SL: Acute and chronic suppression of the central ghrelin signaling system reveals a role in food anticipatory activity. Eur Neuropsychopharmacol 2011;21:384–392.
41 Merkestein M, Brans MA, Luijendijk MC, de Jong JW, Egecioglu E, Dickson SL, Adan RA: Ghrelin mediates anticipation to a palatable meal in rats. Obesity (Silver Spring) 2012;20:963–971.
42 Malik S, McGlone F, Bedrossian D, Dagher A: Ghrelin modulates brain activity in areas that control appetitive behavior. Cell Metab 2008;7:400–409.

43 Roa J, García-Galiano D, Castellano JM, Gaytan F, Pinilla L, Tena-Sempere M: Metabolic control of puberty onset: new players, new mechanisms. Mol Cell Endocrinol 2010;324:87–94.
44 Shah SN, Nyby JG: Ghrelin's quick inhibition of androgen-dependent behaviors of male house mice (*Mus musculus*). Horm Behav 2010;57:291–296.
45 Caquineau C, Leng G, Douglas AJ: Sexual behaviour and neuronal activation in the vomeronasal pathway and hypothalamus of food-deprived male rats. J Neuroendocrinol 2012;24:712–723.
46 Bertoldi ML, Luque EM, Carlini VP, Vincenti LM, Stutz G, Santillán ME, Ruiz RD, Fiol de Cuneo M, Martini AC: Inhibitory effects of ghrelin on sexual behavior: role of the peptide in the receptivity reduction induced by food restriction in mice. Horm Metab Res 2011;43:494–499.
47 Jerlhag E, Egecioglu E, Landgren S, Salomé N, Heilig M, Moechars D, Datta R, Perrissoud D, Dickson SL, Engel JA: Requirement of central ghrelin signaling for alcohol reward. Proc Natl Acad Sci USA 2009; 106:11318–11323.
48 Jerlhag E, Engel JA: Ghrelin receptor antagonism attenuates nicotine-induced locomotor stimulation, accumbal dopamine release and conditioned place preference in mice. Drug Alcohol Depend 2011;117: 126–131.
49 Jerlhag E, Egecioglu E, Dickson SL, Engel JA: Ghrelin receptor antagonism attenuates cocaine- and amphetamine-induced locomotor stimulation, accumbal dopamine release, and conditioned place preference. Psychopharmacology 2010;211:415–422.
50 Jerlhag E: Systemic administration of ghrelin induces conditioned place preference and stimulates accumbal dopamine. Addict Biol 2008;13:358–363.
51 Cummings DE, Weigle DS, Frayo RS, Breen PA, Ma MK, Dellinger EP, Purnell JQ: Plasma ghrelin levels after diet-induced weight loss or gastric bypass surgery. N Engl J Med 2002;346:1623–1630.
52 Briggs DI, Enriori PJ, Lemus MB, Cowley MA, Andrews ZB: Diet-induced obesity causes ghrelin resistance in arcuate NPY/AgRP neurons. Endocrinology 2010;151:4745–4755.
53 Finger BC, Dinan TG, Cryan JF: Diet-induced obesity blunts the behavioural effects of ghrelin: studies in a mouse-progressive ratio task. Psychopharmacology (Berl) 2012;220:173–181.

John R.W. Menzies
Centre for Integrative Physiology
School of Biomedical Sciences, University of Edinburgh
Edinburgh, EH8 9XD (UK)
E-Mail john.menzies@ed.ac.uk

Benso A, Casanueva FF, Ghigo E, Granata A (eds): The Ghrelin System.
Endocr Dev. Basel, Karger, 2013, vol 25, pp 112–121 (DOI: 10.1159/000346059)

Des-Acyl Ghrelin: A Metabolically Active Peptide

Patric J. Delhanty · Sebastian J. Neggers · Aart J. van der Lely
Department of Medicine, Erasmus University MC, Rotterdam, The Netherlands

Abstract

Unacylated ghrelin (UAG), or des-acyl ghrelin, is slowly fighting its way up into the field of interest that studies preproghrelin gene-encoded peptides. Long considered to be an inert degradation product of (acylated) ghrelin (AG), UAG nowadays emerges as an important hormone, separate from the other proghrelin-derived peptides, AG and obestatin. UAG appears to have its own receptor, and it can share this receptor with AG, under experimental conditions at least. An increasing number of studies suggest that UAG can act as a potent functional inhibitor of ghrelin. It can even strongly suppress ghrelin levels in obese human diabetic subjects. Moreover, UAG can improve postprandial glycemia, especially in those subjects in whom preprandial acylated ghrelin levels are high, which makes UAG, or UAG analogs strong potential candidates for the development of drugs for the treatment of metabolic disorders or other conditions in which elevated AG/UAG ratios occur, such as diabetes, obesity and Prader-Willi syndrome.

Since the identification of ghrelin as the ligand of the growth hormone secretagogue receptor type 1a (GHSR-1a) [1] and the realization that ghrelin should be considered as the most potent hunger-inducing hormone, inducing obesity in mice and man, more than 5300 papers have been published on this fascinating peptide (PubMed in early March 2012). The story of unacylated ghrelin (des-acyl ghrelin; UAG) also commenced in 1999, since Kojima et al. [1] described the presence of UAG in the circulation in the same publication in which they described acylated ghrelin. The preproghrelin gene peptides include acylated ghrelin (AG), UAG and obestatin. AGis produced mainly by the stomach and exerts its central and peripheral effects through the GHS-R1a [1]. The ghrelin peptide is acylated by the enzyme ghrelin *O*-acyltransferase, or GOAT [2, 3], which is expressed predominantly in the stomach, gut and pancreas, but also at other sites [4].

The concept that emerged from Kojima's paper and many others was that the ghrelin molecule that lacks the acyl-group, UAG, should be considered as some sort of degradation product without biological activities, as it could not bind and activate the GHSR-1a [1]. Therefore, UAG has never received the level of attention in research and the literature that it deserves, with much less visibility in PubMed than ghrelin, considering the relatively low number of publications (~300 by early March 2012).

However, more and more data are becoming available that strongly suggest that UAG has intrinsic activities in a variety of physiological and pathophysiological situations that are independent of ghrelin itself. These actions sometimes antagonize and sometimes support ghrelin activities.

This chapter tries to address these actions of UAG on metabolism. We describe the properties of UAG in which it seems to act as a functional antagonist of AG. We also describe the newest findings that demonstrate a unique property of UAG, in which it seems to be a strong inhibitor of AG serum levels in vivo in animals and men. Finally, we will address UAG actions in which it behaves as a factor that works independently of AG, characterized by changes in the absence of AG or its receptor GHSR-1a.

Unacylated Ghrelin Is a Functional Ghrelin Antagonist

The first change in paradigm that suggests that UAG should be considered as a separate hormone was reported by Broglio et al. [5] and others (e.g. [6]).

Broglio et al. [5] studied the interaction of the combined administration of AG and UAG in 6 normal young volunteers. As expected, AG markedly increased circulating growth hormone, prolactin, adrenocorticotropin and cortisol levels. AG administration was also followed by a decrease in insulin levels and an increase in plasma glucose levels. UAG alone had no effects. However, when UAG was coadministered with AG, the insulin and glucose response to AG was diminished by UAG. Their findings indicated for the first time that UAG can be metabolically active and can counteract AG actions on at least insulin secretion and glucose metabolism.

Results like these induced some basic research lines that provided more evidence that UAG is a functional ghrelin antagonist. Especially Granata et al. [7] and Delhanty and van der Lely [8] have published good reviews on this topic.

Granata et al. [7] investigated the role of AG in pancreatic β-cell proliferation and apoptosis induced by serum starvation or cytokine (interferon-γ/TNF-α) treatment. β-Cells express AG but not the ghrelin GHSR-1a receptor. However, both UAG and AG recognized common high-affinity binding sites on these cells. Furthermore, both AG and UAG stimulated insulin secretion from HIT-T15 cells. Finally, they both induced cell survival and protection against apoptosis in isolated human islets of Langerhans. These expressed the GHSR-1a receptor, but also expressed separate UAG- and AG-binding sites. So taken together, these data demonstrated that AG and UAG promote survival of human pancreatic β-cells. These effects were found to be independent of the presence of the GHSR-1a receptor, and are likely mediated by specific AG/UAG-binding sites [9].

Another indication that UAG acts as an AG antagonist was demonstrated by Gauna et al. [10]. These authors found that AG stimulates, whereas UAG inhibits glucose output by primary hepatocytes. They studied glucose output by primary porcine hepatocytes in suspension culture, after incubation with AG, UAG, and hexarelin (a GHS-R1a agonist). It was observed that AG dose-dependently induced a glucose output after 20 min of incubation, whereas hexarelin had no effect. In contrast, UAG dose-dependently inhibited glucose release. Moreover, UAG completely reversed AG-induced glucose output. Interestingly, no GHS-R1a gene expression was detectable in the hepatocyte preparations. The observed lack of efficacy of hexarelin, in combination with the efficacy of UAG, and the absence of GHS-R1a expression again indicate the involvement of an uncharacterized ghrelin receptor (sub)type.

Kumar et al. [11] also reported the antagonistic properties of UAG on AG.

Using isolated mouse pancreatic islets they studied the suppression of the spontaneous secretion of pancreatic polypeptide (PP) by AG and obestatin. Interestingly, the PP-releasing effect of AG, but not that of obestatin, was counteracted by UAG. Their results support the view that AG (and obestatin) inhibit spontaneous PP secretion at physiologically relevant concentrations and that they act on separate receptors. However, their results also strongly suggest that UAG acts as a potent inhibitor of AG.

Although the previous observations were all made in in vitro studies, similar observations have been made in rodents, and even in studies in humans.

Further Evidence of the Antagonistic Effect of UAG on Ghrelin

In 2005, Asakawa et al. [12] reported the results of a study in which they examined the effects of UAG on energy balance, by measuring food intake, gastric emptying, c-Fos expression in the hypothalamus, and gene expression of hypothalamic neuropeptides in mice after administration of UAG. Administration of UAG appeared to decrease food intake and gastric emptying rate through actions on the hypothalamus. These antagonistic effects of UAG on AG activity at the central level have been confirmed in elegant studies by Inhoff et al. [13]. These authors investigated the interaction between AG and UAG administered intraperitoneally on food intake and neuronal activity (c-Fos expression) in the arcuate nucleus in nonfasted rats. They found that UAG alone had no effect on food intake. However, the stimulatory effect of AG on food intake was blocked by the coadminstration of UAG. This was reflected in the arcuate nucleus, where UAG significantly reduced the activation of nesfatin-1 immunoreactive neurons by AG when the peptides were coadministered.

To explore the effects of long-term exposure to raised levels of UAG, Asakawa et al. [12] created transgenic mice that overexpressed UAG. UAG transgenic mice exhibited a decrease in body weight, food intake, and fat pad mass accompanied by moderately decreased linear growth, along with a decrease in gastric emptying. Their findings again indicate, but now in vivo, that in contrast to AG, UAG induces negative energy balance by decreasing food intake and delaying gastric emptying.

Following on from the study of Asakawa et al. [12], Zhang et al. [14] studied the effects on adiposity and glucose metabolism of overexpressing UAG in the fat depots of mice, using the fatty acid-binding protein-4 (FABP4) promoter to drive expression of a murine preproghrelin transgene. Circulating UAG levels were significantly higher in FABP4-ghrelin transgenic mice, while no significant change was observed for plasma AG and obestatin. In the presence of high UAG levels, epididymal and perirenal fat masses decreased. FABP4-ghrelin transgenic mice appeared to be resistant to obesity induced by high-fat diet. Brown fat mass, however, was not affected by overexpression of UAG in adipose tissue. Glucose-tolerance tests showed significantly faster clearance of glucose in FABP4-ghrelin transgenic mice than in controls. Insulin-sensitivity testing showed that FABP4-ghrelin transgenic mice had a significantly greater hypoglycemic response to insulin, indicating markedly improved insulin sensitivity [14]. Interestingly, recent evidence suggests that FABP4 promoter is also active in the hypothalamus [15], therefore it is possible that FABP4-ghrelin transgenic mice overexpress UAG at this central site, and that part of the effect may be through antagonism of the actions of AG at a central level.

Unacylated Ghrelin Is a Functional Ghrelin Antagonist, Also in Humans

Several studies have indicated that obese mice and humans seem to have lower UAG levels than normal weight subjects whereas AG levels are similar, indicating that obesity might reflect a relative UAG deficiency, and that UAG levels are regulated by body weight [16–18].

Moreover, insulin-resistant obese subjects have an elevated AG/UAG ratio when compared to insulin-sensitive obese subjects [19, 20].

Ozcan et al. [pers. data] have performed a clinical study on the effects of a continuous overnight infusion of two doses of UAG (3 and 10 μg UAG/kg·h^{-1}) versus placebo in a double-blind crossover study on AG concentrations, and the glucose and insulin responses to a standard breakfast meal (SBM) in 8 overweight patients with controlled type 2 diabetes.

Early morning AG levels (during the overnight infusion, just before the SBM) dropped significantly in the presence of UAG infusions. UAG infusion also markedly decreased AG levels following breakfast.

Moreover, overnight infusions of UAG significantly decreased glucose response to SBM as assessed by continuous glucose monitoring (CGMS), as well as peak serum glucose levels. More striking was the finding of a strong correlation between fasting

AG levels and the amount of postprandial decrease in glucose concentrations during continuous infusion of UAG, using the CGM. The higher the fasting AG levels, the more pronounced the decrease in glucose levels.

This close correlation between the effect of UAG infusion on postprandial glycemia and the preprandial AG levels clearly suggest a potential clinical benefit of UAG administration in especially those subjects in whom relatively high levels of AG can be found. Interesting populations of subjects to study might be those with Prader-Willi syndrome [21, 22] or (subgroups of) patients with metabolic syndrome, especially as there are reports that suggest that diabetes and obesity are linked to a relative UAG deficiency, or increased ratio of AG/UAG blood levels [13, 23–25]. The potential clinical importance of inhibiting AG has been reported before in rodents. Barnett et al. [26] reported the design, synthesis and characterization of GO-CoA-Tat, a peptide-based bisubstrate analog that antagonizes GOAT. With this compound, they observed that the intraperitoneal administration of GO-CoA-Tat improved glucose tolerance and reduced weight gain in wild-type mice. Interestingly, they did not observe this reduction in weight gain in ghrelin-deficient mice that lack both AG and UAG. This might suggest that these animals respond less well to GO-CoA-TAT treatment because they are UAG deficient [26].

Another report by Maletinska et al. [27] on the potential beneficial effects of antagonizing AG showed that the ghrelin receptor antagonist [D-Lys(3)] GHRP-6, after seven days of subcutaneous treatment, markedly decreased food intake in ovariectomized mice fed both high-fat and standard diets. Furthermore, this AG antagonist reduced body weight, blood glucose, insulin and leptin.

The concept that high UAG over AG ratios are accompanied by an improved metabolic state was supported by Cederberg et al. [28], who found that in 552 young men undergoing military service an increase in UAG after 6 months of an intensive long-term exercise intervention was associated with improvements in body weight and body composition.

This is in line with a recent report by Benso et al. [29] in which they showed that overnight infusions of UAG improved postprandial glycemia without increasing insulin levels, suggesting a potent insulin sensitizing effect of UAG.

GHSR-1a Independent Effects of UAG

It might seem obvious to the reader that UAG must have GHSR-1a independent effects, since Kojima et al. [1] reported that UAG does not bind to the GHSR-1a in their paper on the discovery of ghrelin.

However, Gauna et al. [30] reported that UAG was found to be a full agonist of the GHSR-1a with an EC_{50} of between 1.6 and 2 nM using an in vitro system. Correspondingly, UAG displaced radiolabeled AG from the GHSR-1a with an IC_{50} of 13 nM. In addition, GHSR-1a antagonists were found to block UAG induced changes with approximately similar potency to their effect on ghrelin activation of the GHSR-1a, suggesting a similar mode of action. These findings demonstrate that in a defined system UAG does not antagonize activation of the GHSR-1a by AG. Moreover, this finding also emphasizes the importance of assessing the concentration of UAG used in both in vitro and in vivo experimental systems that are aimed at examining GHSR-1a independent effects.

Delhanty and van der Lely [8] tried to address just these GHSR-1a-independent effects of UAG in a study in mice in which they assessed potential mechanisms of UAG action in vivo. They examined rapid effects of UAG on genomewide expression patterns in fat, muscle and liver of GHSR-1a ablated mice using microarrays. The obtained expression data were analyzed using ingenuity pathways analysis and gene set enrichment analysis. Regulation of subsets of these genes was verified by quantitative PCR in independent experiments. They found that UAG acutely regulated clusters of genes involved in glucose and lipid metabolism in all three tissues, consistent with enhancement of insulin sensitivity. This pivotal set of studies demonstrates that UAG rapidly modulates the expression of metabolically important genes in these tissues, which are central to the control of lipid and glucose homeostasis. As the studies were done in GHSR-deleted mice, these results strongly indicate a direct, GHSR-1a independent, action of UAG that improves insulin sensitivity and metabolic profile.

As already addressed earlier in this chapter, the group of Granata et al. [9] described that both UAG and AG recognized common high-affinity binding sites on pancreatic β-cells, separate from the binding of AG to the GHSR-1a receptor. AG and UAG activated phosphatidylinositol 3-kinase (PI3K)/Akt and ERK1/2, whereas PI3K and MAPK inhibitors counteracted the ghrelin antiapoptotic effect. Furthermore, both AG and UAG stimulated insulin secretion from HIT-T15 cells, which express the GHSR-1a. Again, both AG and UAG caused proliferation and protection against apoptosis through identical signaling pathways. On top of that, both peptides inhibited cytokine-induced NO increase in both HIT-T15 and INS-1E cells. Finally, both AG- and UAG-induced cell survival and protected human islets of Langerhans cells against apoptosis. These human islets of Langerhans expressed the GHSR-1a, but also showed other UAG- and AG-binding sites. Their data suggest that AG and UAG can both promote survival of β-cells in human islets.

Gauna et al. [31] investigated the interactions between AG and UAG on ghrelin receptors in INS-1E rat insulinoma cells, using insulin secretion after 30 min static incubation as a read-out. A possible involvement of the GHS-R1a as a putative receptor for UAG was also studied by determining its mRNA expression and the functional effects of GHSR-1a antagonists on insulin release. It was observed that both UAG and AG dose-dependently stimulated insulin release in the nanomolar range. The AG-induced insulin output was antagonized by two GHS-R1a antagonists ([D-Lys(3)]GHRP-6 and BIM28163), which did not block UAG actions. These effects occurred in the presence of low levels of GHSR-1a mRNA. Their data support the

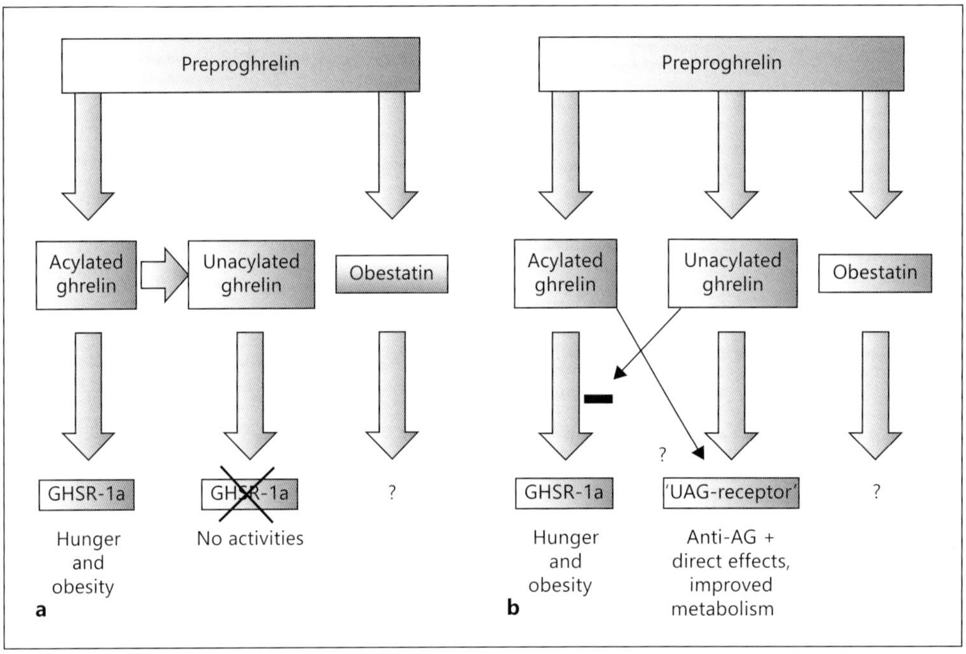

Fig. 1. a The old paradigm, in which UAG is considered to be 'just' a degradation product of AG, without any activity, not able to bind to a receptor. **b** The proposed new paradigm of the physiological role of UAG, using its own, yet identified, receptor, that can probably also bind AG. UAG is also a functional antagonist of AG.

existence of a specific receptor for UAG, other than the GHS-R1a, that it can share with AG.

Halem et al. [32] in 2005 also reported on the potential presence of a non-GHSR-1a receptor. They demonstrated that BIM-28163 blocked AG activation of the GHSR-1a receptor, and inhibited AG-induced GH secretion in vivo. However, BIM-28163 also acted as an agonist with regard to stimulating weight gain. These results may suggest the presence of an unknown ghrelin receptor that modulates ghrelin actions on weight gain. Moreover, BIM-28163 acted as an antagonist of AG-induced Fos protein immunoreactivity (Fos-IR) in the medial arcuate nucleus, an area involved in the AG modulation of GH secretion. However, in the dorsal medial hypothalamus (DMH), a region associated with regulation of food intake, both AG and BIM-28163 acted as agonists that upregulated Fos-IR. Their observation that AG and BIM-28163 have different efficacies in inducing Fos-IR in the DMH, and that concomitant administration of AG and an excess of BIM-28163 resulted in the same level of Fos-IR as BIM-28163 administered alone may demonstrate that in the DMH both AG and BIM-28163 act via the same receptor. If so, it is unlikely that this receptor is GHSR-1a. Most importantly, this might imply that GHSR-1a may not be the most appropriate target for anti-obesity strategies.

Without knowing which receptor transduces the UAG signal (and sometimes also the GHSR-1a independent AG signal) to cells and tissues, it is difficult to predict how GHSR-1a blocking agents will affect, for example, metabolism and apoptosis. This is particularly pertinent in tissues such as the pancreas where UAG and AG work together to promote cell survival and protect against cytokine-induced cell death.

Therefore, we suggest a new paradigm for the role of AG and UAG in (patho) physiology, as depicted in figure 1. While figure 1a shows the old paradigm, figure 1b shows the proposed role of UAG, using its own, as yet unidentified, receptor that can probably also bind AG. UAG is also a functional antagonist of AG.

In conclusion, UAG is becoming more and more recognized as a separate hormone, with its own actions, independent from the actions of AG. Mostly, it antagonizes but sometimes it works together with AG. Although UAG can bind and activate the AG receptor, it does not reach the necessary concentrations in tissues to do so, at least under physiological conditions and perhaps even in the presence of pharmacological levels of UAG. Therefore, the low affinity of the GHSR-1a for UAG excludes this receptor as a mediator for the growing number of observations of UAG activity in vitro and in vivo.

The fact that increased AG/UAG levels are linked to obesity and diabetes, and that UAG administration induces a rapid decrease in circulating AG levels, along with an improvement in glycemic control, might open ways to use UAG or UAG analogues to combat these conditions.

References

1 Kojima M, Hosoda H, Date Y, Nakazato M, Matsuo H, Kangawa K: Ghrelin is a growth-hormone-releasing acylated peptide from stomach. Nature 1999;402: 656–660.

2 Gutierrez JA, Solenberg PJ, Perkins DR, Willency JA, Knierman MD, Jin Z, Witcher DR, Luo S, Onyia JE, Hale JE: Ghrelin octanoylation mediated by an orphan lipid transferase. Proc Natl Acad Sci USA 2008; 105:6320–6325.

3 Yang J, Brown MS, Liang G, Grishin NV, Goldstein JL: Identification of the acyltransferase that octanoylates ghrelin, an appetite-stimulating peptide hormone. Cell 2008;132:387–396.

4 Kang K, Schmahl J, Lee JM, Garcia K, Patil K, Chen A, Keene M, Murphy A, Sleeman MW: Mouse ghrelin-O-acyltransferase (GOAT) plays a critical role in bile acid reabsorption. FASEB J 2012;26:259–271.

5 Broglio F, Gottero C, Prodam F, Gauna C, Muccioli G, Papotti M, Abribat T, van der Lely AJ, Ghigo E: Non-acylated ghrelin counteracts the metabolic but not the neuroendocrine response to acylated ghrelin in humans. J Clin Endocrinol Metab 2004;89:3062–3065.

6 Gauna C, Meyler FM, Janssen J, Delhanty PJD, Abribat T, Van Koetsveld P, Hofland LJ, Broglio F, Ghigo E, van der Lely AJ: Administration of acylated ghrelin reduces insulin sensitivity, whereas the combination of acylated plus unacylated ghrelin strongly improves insulin sensitivity. J Clin Endocrinol Metab 2004;89:5035–5042.

7 Granata R, Baragli A, Settanni F, Scarlatti F, Ghigo E: Unraveling the role of the ghrelin gene peptides in the endocrine pancreas. J Mol Endocrinol 2010;45: 107–118.

8 Delhanty PJ, van der Lely AJ: Ghrelin and glucose homeostasis. Peptides 2011;32:2309–2318.

9 Granata R, Settanni F, Biancone L, Trovato L, Nano R, Bertuzzi F, Destefanis S, Annunziata M, Martinetti M, Catapano F, Ghe C, Isgaard J, Papotti M, Ghigo E, Muccioli G: Acylated and unacylated ghrelin promote proliferation and inhibit apoptosis of pancreatic beta-cells and human islets: involvement of 3′,5′-cyclic adenosine monophosphate/protein kinase A, extracellular signal-regulated kinase 1/2, and phosphatidylinositol 3-kinase/Akt signaling. Endocrinology 2007;148:512–529.
10 Gauna C, Delhanty PJ, Hofland LJ, Janssen JA, Broglio F, Ross RJ, Ghigo E, van der Lely AJ: Ghrelin stimulates, whereas des-octanoyl ghrelin inhibits, glucose output by primary hepatocytes. J Clin Endocrinol Metab 2005;90:1055–1060.
11 Kumar R, Salehi A, Rehfeld JF, Hoglund P, Lindstrom E, Hakanson R: Proghrelin peptides: Desacyl ghrelin is a powerful inhibitor of acylated ghrelin, likely to impair physiological effects of acyl ghrelin but not of obestatin. A study of pancreatic polypeptide secretion from mouse islets. Regul Pept 2010; 164:65–70.
12 Asakawa A, Inui A, Fujimiya M, Sakamaki R, Shinfuku N, Ueta Y, Meguid MM, Kasuga M: Stomach regulates energy balance via acylated ghrelin and desacyl ghrelin. Gut 2005;54:18–24.
13 Inhoff T, Monnikes H, Noetzel S, Stengel A, Goebel M, Dinh QT, Riedl A, Bannert N, Wisser AS, Wiedenmann B, Klapp BF, Tache Y, Kobelt P: Desacyl ghrelin inhibits the orexigenic effect of peripherally injected ghrelin in rats. Peptides 2008;29:2159–2168.
14 Zhang W, Chai B, Li JY, Wang H, Mulholland MW: Effect of des-acyl ghrelin on adiposity and glucose metabolism. Endocrinology 2008;149:4710–4716.
15 Martens K, Bottelbergs A, Baes M: Ectopic recombination in the central and peripheral nervous system by aP2/FABP4-Cre mice: implications for metabolism research. FEBS Lett 2010;584:1054–1058.
16 Longo KA, Charoenthongtrakul S, Giuliana DJ, Govek EK, McDonagh T, Qi Y, DiStefano PS, Geddes BJ: Improved insulin sensitivity and metabolic flexibility in ghrelin receptor knockout mice. Regul Pept 2008; 150:55–61.
17 Nonogaki K, Nozue K, Oka Y: Hyperphagia alters expression of hypothalamic 5-HT2C and 5-HT1B receptor genes and plasma des-acyl ghrelin levels in Ay mice. Endocrinology 2006;147:5893–900.
18 Pacifico L, Poggiogalle E, Costantino F, Anania C, Ferraro F, Chiarelli F, Chiesa C: Acylated and nonacylated ghrelin levels and their associations with insulin resistance in obese and normal weight children with metabolic syndrome. Eur J Endocrinol 2009; 161:861–870.
19 St-Pierre DH, Karelis AD, Coderre L, Malita F, Fontaine J, Mignault D, Brochu M, Bastard JP, Cianflone K, Doucet E, Imbeault P, Rabasa-Lhoret R: Association of acylated and nonacylated ghrelin with insulin sensitivity in overweight and obese postmenopausal women. J Clin Endocrinol Metab 2007;92:264–269.
20 Barazzoni R, Zanetti M, Ferreira C, Vinci P, Pirulli A, Mucci M, Dore F, Fonda M, Ciocchi B, Cattin L, Guarnieri G: Relationships between desacylated and acylated ghrelin and insulin sensitivity in the metabolic syndrome. J Clin Endocrinol Metab 2007;92: 3935–3940.
21 Prodam F, Bellone S, Grugni G, Crino A, Ragusa L, Franzese A, Di Battista E, Corrias A, Walker G, Rapa A, Aimaretti G, Bona G: Influence of age, gender, and glucose tolerance on fasting and fed acylated ghrelin in Prader-Willi syndrome. Clin Nutr 2009; 28:94–99.
22 Yi CX, Heppner K, Tschop MH: Ghrelin in eating disorders. Mol Cell Endocrinol 2011;340:29–34.
23 Miegueu P, St Pierre D, Broglio F, Cianflone K: Effect of desacyl ghrelin, obestatin and related peptides on triglyceride storage, metabolism and GHSR signaling in 3T3-L1 adipocytes. J Cell Biochem 2011;112: 704–714.
24 Mackelvie KJ, Meneilly GS, Elahi D, Wong AC, Barr SI, Chanoine JP: Regulation of appetite in lean and obese adolescents after exercise: role of acylated and desacyl ghrelin. J Clin Endocrinol Metab 2007;92: 648–654.
25 Kim HJ, Lee S, Kim TW, Kim HH, Jeon TY, Yoon YS, Oh SW, Kwak H, Lee JG: Effects of exercise-induced weight loss on acylated and unacylated ghrelin in overweight children. Clin Endocrinol (Oxf) 2008; 68:416–422.
26 Barnett BP, Hwang Y, Taylor MS, Kirchner H, Pfluger PT, Bernard V, Lin YY, Bowers EM, Mukherjee C, Song WJ, Longo PA, Leahy DJ, Hussain MA, Tschop MH, Boeke JD, Cole PA: Glucose and weight control in mice with a designed ghrelin *O*-acyltransferase inhibitor. Science 2010;330:1689–1692.
27 Maletinska L, Matyskova R, Maixnerova J, Sykora D, Pychova M, Spolcova A, Blechova M, Drapalova J, Lacinova Z, Haluzik M, Zelezna B: The Peptidic GHS-R antagonist [D-Lys(3)]GHRP-6 markedly improves adiposity and related metabolic abnormalities in a mouse model of postmenopausal obesity. Mol Cell Endocrinol 2011;343:55–62.
28 Cederberg H, Rajala U, Koivisto VM, Jokelainen J, Surcel HM, Keinanen-Kiukaanniemi S, Laakso M: Unacylated ghrelin is associated with changes in body composition and body fat distribution during long-term exercise intervention. Eur J Endocrinol. 2011;165:243–248.

29 Benso A, St-Pierre D, Prodam F, Gramaglia E, Granata R, Van der Lely AJ, Ghigo E, Broglio F: Metabolic effects of overnight continuous infusion of unacylated ghrelin in humans. Eur J Endocrinol 2012;166:911–916.
30 Gauna C, van de ZB, van KA, Themmen AP, van der Lely AJ, Delhanty PJ: Unacylated ghrelin is not a functional antagonist but a full agonist of the type 1a growth hormone secretagogue receptor (GHS-R). Mol Cell Endocrinol 2007;274:30–34.
31 Gauna C, Delhanty PJ, van Aken MO, Janssen JA, Themmen AP, Hofland LJ, Culler M, Broglio F, Ghigo E, van der Lely AJ: Unacylated ghrelin is active on the INS-1E rat insulinoma cell line independently of the growth hormone secretagogue receptor type 1a and the corticotropin releasing factor 2 receptor. Mol Cell Endocrinol 2006;251:103–111.
32 Halem HA, Taylor JE, Dong JZ, Shen Y, Datta R, Abizaid A, Diano S, Horvath TL, Culler MD: A novel growth hormone secretagogue-1a receptor antagonist that blocks ghrelin-induced growth hormone secretion but induces increased body weight gain. Neuroendocrinology 2005;81:339–349.

Prof. Aart J. van der Lely, MD, PhD
Head of Endocrinology, Erasmus University MC
PO Box 2040
NL–3000 CA Rotterdam (The Netherlands)
E-Mail a.vanderlelij@erasmusmc.nl

Benso A, Casanueva FF, Ghigo E, Granata A (eds): The Ghrelin System.
Endocr Dev. Basel, Karger, 2013, vol 25, pp 122–134 (DOI: 10.1159/000346061)

Ghrelin and Tumors

Mauro Papotti · Eleonora Duregon · Marco Volante
Department of Clinical and Biological Sciences, University of Turin at San Luigi Hospital, Orbassano, Turin, Italy

Abstract
Since the original discovery of ghrelin and, subsequently, obestatin (the alternative product of the ghrelin gene), a major interest has been devoted to the investigation of their central and peripheral activities in physiological conditions as well as on their role in metabolic diseases. However, several studies with different methodological approaches variably identified ghrelin and obestatin synthesis and secretion in several neoplastic conditions, including neuroendocrine and non-neuroendocrine cancers of various sites. Moreover, in vitro studies showed the capability of ghrelin to modulate tumor cell functions such as cell proliferation, apoptosis and invasiveness, although with variable and even paradoxical effects in different cell models. Interestingly, in most studies, it was demonstrated that ghrelin exerts its pro- or antineoplastic properties by means of receptors other than GHSR1a, that still need to be identified. However, the possible usefulness of the modulation of the ghrelin/obestatin axis in neoplastic conditions using either synthetic agonists or antagonists, though interesting in perspective, is still far from clinical applicability, and probably more related to the regulation of specific metabolic pathways in tumor cells, including lipid and carbohydrate use, than to the specific modulation of cell proliferation.

Ghrelin and obestatin are, respectively, 28 and 23 amino acid peptide hormones, which derive from the processing of the same pre-pro-ghrelin precursor coded by the ghrelin gene (GHRL). Ghrelin was originally discovered in the gastric mucosa [1], but it was demonstrated in a wide range of normal and tumoral tissues. It can exist in two forms, acylated and nonacylated, and acylation is mediated by the ghrelin O-acyltransferase (GOAT) enzyme. Acylated ghrelin is the natural ligand of the only currently known ghrelin receptor, the growth hormone secretagogue receptor (GHSR) type 1a. To date, the acyl-ghrelin/GHSR1a system has been directly associated with multiple physiological functions related to the regulation of energy balance and metabolic function at the central and peripheral levels. However, ghrelin and its receptor are also present in many endocrine and nonendocrine tumors (for example, gastro-entero-pancreatic, pituitary, prostate, breast), and in corresponding cancer cell line models where ghrelin has been shown to control neoplastic cell proliferation, apoptosis and migration. Yet, the precise role of the ghrelin system in cancer is poorly understood. As an example, a truncated isoform of GHSR1a, the GHSR type 1b, has been found in the majority of the tumors and cancer cell lines cited above, but its potential role in tumor regulation remains unknown. The alternative product of the ghrelin gene, obestatin, was originally reported to be the ligand for the orphan G protein-coupled receptor 39 (GPR39). However, as several groups were unable to confirm that obestatin has agonist properties on GPR39 or activates specific GPR39 signaling, a specific obestatin receptor remains unknown, to date. Like ghrelin, obestatin can be expressed in both normal and tumoral tissues and there is a growing evidence that both hormones play an autocrine/paracrine role in a number of processes related to cancer progression, including cell proliferation, cell migration, and apoptosis, possibly acting with opposed mechanisms. Nevertheless, information about any prognostic role of both hormones is still scant.

From a methodological standpoint, ghrelin, obestatin and GHSR can be detected at both gene and protein levels by means of in situ hybridization, Northern blotting or reverse transcriptase-polymerase chain reaction (RT-PCR) and immunohistochemistry (IHC). However, since all of them have been widely reported in normal cells and tissues, including blood vessels, their demonstration in a tumor cell population needs specific cellular localization of the mRNA/protein by means of in situ hybridization or IHC. Ghrelin-binding sites have been known for several years, even before the identification of this hormone, since GHSR were previously known to be bound by synthetic peptides called growth hormone secretagogues (GHS) that share with ghrelin a similar affinity profile. However, studies combining the displacement capacity of radiolabeled synthetic peptidyl GHS ([^{125}I]Tyr-Ala-hexarelin) and GHSR1a mRNA analysis suggested that some normal and tumor tissues bind ghrelin and synthetic GHS, but lack GHSR1a, thus supporting that other receptor subtypes may be also present. All data summarized herein, with special reference to those related to the tissue expression of the hormones and receptors, are highly heterogeneous in terms of methodology applied, and the alternative techniques might be responsible for some of the controversies still pending on this issue.

Ghrelin and its Receptors in Tumors (table 1)

Ghrelin and Its Receptors in Endocrine Tumors

Gastro-Entero-Pancreatic Neuroendocrine Neoplasms (NENs). Most of the data available so far are related to well-differentiated gastric NENs. In these tumors, ghrelin has been demonstrated in a relatively high percentage of cases (12/16, 25/33 and 12/20 in three series; see Vu et al. [2] for review), accounting for a total of 75% of cases by means of IHC (fig. 1) and 81% by means of ISH, with a 94% concordance between the two procedures. Most of these cases were associated with chronic atrophic gastritis

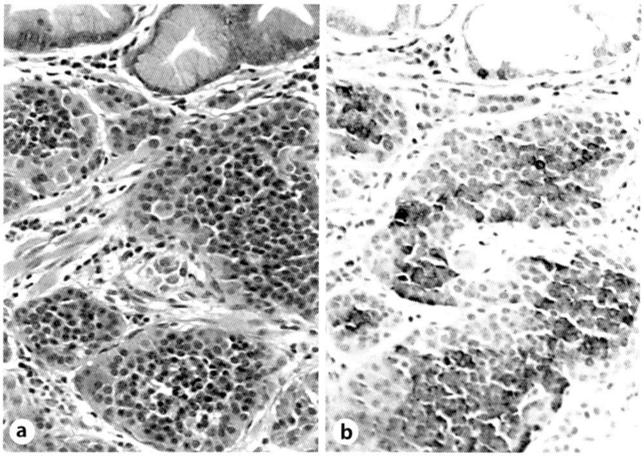

Fig. 1. A case of well-differentiated neuroendocrine tumor of the stomach (**a**) with a diffuse expression of ghrelin protein (**b**); isolated neuroendocrine cells of the normal gastric mucosa (**b**, top of figure) are also immunoreactive. **a** HE. **b** Immunoperoxidase. **a**, **b** Original magnification ×200.

Table 1. Tumors in which significant ghrelin expression has been reported

Organ	Tumor type	Additional comment
Gastro-intestinal tract	NE gastric tumors	ECL cell tumor type
	NE intestinal tumors	decreasing prevalence from ileum to colon
	gastric adenocarcinoma	–
	colorectal adenocarcinoma	positive correlation with high tumor stage
	esophageal adenocarcinoma	–
	GIST	–
Pancreas	NE tumors	no association with other hormones
Lung	carcinoids	focal protein expression
Thyroid	follicular cell-derived tumors	stronger in malignant tumors
	medullary carcinoma	–
Pituitary	adenomas	stronger in somatotroph and nonfunctioning adenomas
Adrenal	adrenocortical adenomas	stronger in cortisol secreting adenomas
Testis	Leydig cell tumor	–
Prostate	adenocarcinoma	expression of exon 3-deleted pre-pro-ghrelin
Breast	invasive carcinoma	prognostic impact; expression of exon 3-deleted and In1-ghrelin variants
Endometrium	endometrioid carcinoma	controversial

NE = Neuroendocrine.

and were probably of entero-chromaffin-like (ECL) type, as commonly observed in this location. Although the putative ghrelin producing cell of the stomach is the X/A like cell, the corresponding endocrine tumors are exceedingly rare and it is likely that ghrelin is 'ectopically' expressed by conventional ECL carcinoids. The extent of ghrelin expression was either focal or diffuse and peritumoral hyperplastic endocrine cells (in the context of atrophic gastritis) were also intensely expressing ghrelin. Antral carcinoids were generally unreactive, as well as the cases of poorly differentiated NENs analyzed so far. In parallel with the decreased number of ghrelin producing cells in the small and large intestine as compared to the stomach, intestinal NENs produce ghrelin in a smaller fraction of cases.

Well-differentiated pancreatic NENs were also found to express ghrelin in variable percentages, ranging from 25 to 81% [3, 4]. The presence of ghrelin in pancreatic NETs is not surprising, since several groups documented the presence of ghrelin in fetal and adult islets of Langerhans. Although discrepant data appeared in the literature regarding the cell type producing ghrelin, its production was observed in insulinomas, glucagonomas, gastrinomas and somatostatinomas as well as in clinically not functioning tumors [4, 5]. Ghrelin expression has been shown also in multiple endocrine neoplasia type 1 (MEN-1) associated tumors, with variable rates according to the site of involvement and different studies. In total, only 2 cases of gastric and pancreatic NETs have been reported in the literature as 'ghrelinomas', based on extremely high levels of circulating ghrelin and vague clinical symptoms, including body mass index preservation even in advanced stages of the disease.

With regard to ghrelin receptors, variable prevalence of GHSR mRNA expression has been documented in neuroendocrine tumors of different types [6]. Our group analyzed a relatively large series of 42 gastro-entero-pancreatic neuroendocrine tumors [4, 7]. By means of RT-PCR, 14/28 pancreatic endocrine tumors were shown to contain GHS-R 1b mRNA and half of them also contained type 1a transcripts. All GHS-R-positive tumors were insulinomas, while those positive for type 1b included either insulinomas or other functioning and nonfunctioning neoplasms. Of the 14 gastrointestinal NENs examined, 7 were shown to contain GHS-R 1a and/or 1b (all localized in the intestine). All GHS-R-positive NENs also expressed ghrelin mRNA. Ekeblad et al. [5] confirmed the expression of GHS-R in 70% of pancreatic NENs by means of immunohistochemistry.

Lung Neuroendocrine Tumors. In this tumor group, ghrelin immunoreactivity was detected in half of the samples in a single study [3], and ghrelin mRNA was documented in 9/9 typical carcinoids, 2/3 atypical carcinoids and 2/2 small cells lung carcinomas in another [8]. Neuroendocrine tumors of the lung were found to contain also GHS binding sites [9]. Interestingly, in this latter study the comparison between binding experiments using GHS analogs and GHSR mRNA analysis showed that only half of the cases positive with the binding procedure expressed GHSR mRNA, confirming that in the peripheral tissues additional receptors probably exist, other than GHS-R 1a and 1b.

Pituitary Adenomas. Ghrelin mRNA was detected in 93% of the over 100 tumor tested by both RT-PCR and IHC methods [10]. Variable expression of ghrelin was observed in different pituitary adenoma subtypes, since quantitative measurement of ghrelin mRNA showed that ghrelin expression was relatively low in prolactinomas and corticotroph adenomas and relatively high in somatotroph and nonfunctioning adenomas, compared with that of normal pituitary tissue [6, 11]. Ghrelin-binding sites were also detected in the pituitary gland and in the vast majority of tumors so far investigated, regardless of the tumor cell type and hormone produced. Nonfunctioning adenomas were also shown to express GHS-R mRNA by most authors.

Thyroid, Adrenal and Testicular Tumors. Medullary thyroid carcinoma samples and TT cell line were shown to contain ghrelin protein and mRNA [12], but ghrelin plasma levels are not modified in patients with medullary thyroid cancer [13]. In follicular-derived thyroid tumors, ghrelin (but not GHSR1a) is widely expressed, with special reference to malignant ones, but with no apparent differences in different tumor grades [14]. Moreover, in a study detecting GH secretagogue binding sites in benign and malignant human thyroid tumors of follicular origin, the values of binding found in benign tumors were similar to those of nontumoral thyroid parenchyma whereas those in cancer were much higher [15]. The significance of ghrelin production by thyroid tumor cells is poorly understood, but the presence of coexpression of ghrelin and ghrelin-binding sites suggests that the hormone may act directly on the tumor cells using auto/paracrine loops alternative from GHSR.

In adrenal tumors, ghrelin has been documented in cortisol-producing adenomas (87% of cases by means of RT-PCR), whereas adrenocortical carcinomas and pheochromocytomas showed a weak/absent expression of ghrelin at both mRNA and protein levels. GHS-R1a was undetectable in about 60% of both benign and malignant adrenocortical tumor samples, except for cortisol-producing adenomas, which showed increased receptor expression [16].

In the testis, ghrelin and GHSR1a protein and mRNA have been demonstrated in well-differentiated Leydig cell tumors, but not in germ cell neoplasms [17].

Ghrelin and Its Receptors in Nonendocrine Tumors

Ghrelin and ghrelin-binding sites or GHSR have been heterogeneously detected in tumors of nonendocrine type, in parallel with the growing evidence that ghrelin gene products are also expressed/secreted by a widespread subpopulation of nonendocrine cells. In prostate cancer, ghrelin mRNA and protein have been detected in tumor tissues and cell lines, the latter also secreting ghrelin in the culture medium [18]. Extensive ghrelin expression has also been observed in breast cancer tissues. In a recent study, ghrelin (and obestatin) immunoreactivity was determined in 71.5% (and 77.1% for obestatin) of invasive breast cancers, with a correlation with low histological grade, estrogen receptor positivity, small tumor size and low proliferation index. Moreover, ghrelin expression was significantly correlated to better recurrence-free and breast cancer-specific survival at both uni- and multivariate analyses [19]. In addition, specific ghrelin isoforms have been documented in breast cancer tissues, particularly the exon 3-deleted pre-pro-ghrelin [20] and a novel ghrelin variant (which contains Ex0–1, intron 1, and Ex2) encoding a pre-pro-peptide that conserves the first 12 amino acids of native ghrelin, but would have a different C-terminal tail [21].

Both such isoforms are significantly over-expressed in neoplastic as compared to normal breast tissue, but are apparently not correlated with native ghrelin or GHSR1a expression. In endometrial cancer, conflicting results have been reported, ghrelin being found either positive in endometrial cancer tissues and cell lines [22] or consistently negative in malignant as compared to normal/hyperplastic endometrium [23]. The ghrelin axis has also been investigated in gastrointestinal cancer. Ghrelin has been detected in colorectal cancers with special reference to well and moderately differentiated tumors, and positively correlated with high tumor stage. Interestingly, GHSR1b showed the same association, whereas GHSR1a followed an inverse correlation with stage as compared to ghrelin [24]. Moreover, in a case-control study, two single nucleotide polymorphisms of the ghrelin gene GHRL, namely rs27647 and rs35683, have been associated with a lower risk of colorectal cancer development [25]. Ghrelin expression has been also detected in a high percentage of esophageal and gastric adenocarcinomas [26] by means of immunohistochemistry and RT-PCR, as well as in gastrointestinal stromal tumors (GIST) [27]. By contrast, most renal cell tumors (42 cases overall analyzed including clear cell, chromophobe, papillary carcinomas and oncocytomas) studied by means of radioimmunoassay and immunohistochemistry expressed ghrelin to a significantly lower extent than normal kidney [28]. Ghrelin mRNA, but not the protein, has also been detected in non-small cell lung cancer, particularly in 6/12 squamous cell carcinomas and in 10/15 adenocarcinomas [8]. Finally, GHSR1a (but not ghrelin) was investigated in ovarian tumors by means of immunohistochemistry. Similarly to non-neoplastic conditions, benign serous tumors and well-differentiated serous cystoadenocarcinomas were positive, whereas other neoplasms, such as mucinous cystoadenomas and cystoadenocarcinomas, endometrioid tumors, clear cell carcinomas, and Brenner tumors, did not express the receptor GHS-R1a [29].

Obestatin in Tumors (table 2)

Obestatin protein and transcripts have been investigated more recently and less extensively than those of ghrelin. Our group [30] described obestatin expression by means of immunohistochemistry and RT-PCR in a small series (23/105) of endocrine tumors from various sites, including gastric (4/5) and pancreatic (8/22) neuroendocrine neoplasms. Adrenocortical adenomas and carcinomas, pheochromocytomas and neuroendocrine lung tumors were all negative. With the notable exception of single cases of parathyroid and thyroid tumors (both medullary and follicular derived carcinomas), all obestatin-positive tumors had a focal reactivity, with scattered reactive cells within the tumor cell population (fig. 2). In the majority of cases, ghrelin immunoreactivity was observed in the same obestatin-positive tumor areas, usually with a more intense and diffuse pattern of staining. Double immunohistochemical reactions demonstrated that obestatin-positive cells represent a fraction of the ghre-

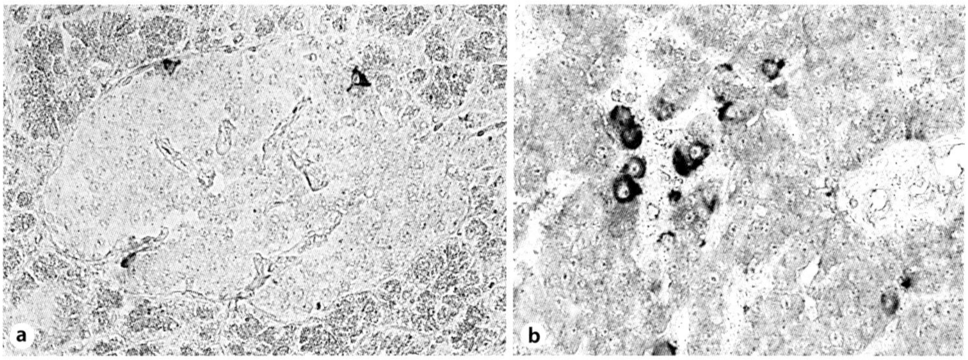

Fig. 2. Obestatin protein expression in rare peripheral cells of a normal pancreatic islet (**a**), and in scattered tumor cells of a well-differentiated neuroendocrine tumor of the pancreas (**b**). **a**, **b** Immunoperoxidase. Original magnification ×250.

Table 2. Tumors in which significant obestatin expression has been reported

Organ	Tumor type	Additional comment
Gastrointestinal tract	NE gastric tumors NE intestinal tumors	scattered positive cells
Pancreas	NE tumors	scattered positive cells, no association with other hormones
Thyroid	follicular cell-derived carcinomas medullary carcinoma	diffuse pattern –
Parathyroid	carcinoma	one single case reported; adenomas negative
Breast	invasive carcinoma	no prognostic impact

NE = Neuroendocrine.

lin-secreting tumor cell population. In another study, 63 gastric endocrine tumors were analyzed by means of immunohistochemistry for ghrelin, obestatin and vesicular monoamine transporter-2 (VMAT-2), a marker of enterochromaffin-like (ECL) cells. Obestatin and ghrelin immunoreactivity always occurred in the same endocrine cells in the gastric mucosa, whereas VMAT-2 was only occasionally co-expressed by these cells, as opposed to what observed in tumors, were the co-expression of obestatin, ghrelin and VMAT-2 was nearly always detected, except for two cases of functioning ghrelin-producing tumors ('ghrelinomas') [31]. In the thyroid, obestatin immunoreactivity was also described by Karaoglu et al. [32], who detected obestatin protein in both papillary thyroid carcinomas and non-neoplastic tissues. They did not find any difference in obestatin levels with regard to the benign or malignant nature of thyroid disease, at variance with previous findings on ghrelin expression [14]. Finally, with regard to nonendocrine tumors, obestatin protein was detected in 77% of 144 breast

Table 3. Ghrelin effects on tumor cell biology

Tumor	Cell line	Biological effect	Ref. no.
Adrenocortical carcinoma	NCI-H295R, SW-13	stimulates proliferation	[16]
	SW-13	stimulates proliferation, antiapoptotic	[38]
	NCI-H295R, SW-13	proapoptotic	[39]
Pancreatic adenocarcinoma	PANC1, MIAPaCa2, BxPC3, Capan2	stimulates proliferation, increases migration	[42]
Colorectal carcinoma	SW-48, RKO	stimulates proliferation, increases migration	[24]
	HT-29	antiapoptotic	[37]
Endometrial carcinoma	Ishikawa, HEC1B, KLE	stimulates proliferation antiapoptotic	[22]
Prostate carcinoma	PC-3, DU 145	stimulates proliferation	[18]
	PC-3	inhibits proliferation, proapoptotic	[34]
	PC-3, LNCaP, DU145	low concentrations stimulates vs. high concentrations inhibits proliferation	[35]
Esophageal adenocarcinoma	OE-19	no role in apoptosis	[40]
Breast carcinoma	T47D, MCF7, MDA-MB-231, MB-435, MCF10A	stimulates proliferation	[20]
	MCF7, MDA-MB 231	inhibits proliferation	[36]
Thyroid carcinoma	ARO, N-PAP	inhibits proliferation	[14]
Small cell lung carcinoma	H345, Calu-1	inhibits proliferation, proapoptotic	[8]
Astrocytoma	U-118, U-87, CCF-STTG1, SW1088	increases migration	[41]

carcinomas (see also above) with a significant association with low histological grade, estrogen receptor positivity, small tumor size and low proliferation index, though not with prognosis [19].

Role of Ghrelin in Cancer Growth Control and Progression (table 3)

The finding that ghrelin and ghrelin/GHS receptors are coexpressed in several tumors and related cell lines suggests that ghrelin is likely to play an important autocrine/paracrine role in neoplastic conditions. By now, three main processes have been investigated: proliferation, apoptosis and migration. It is currently unclear whether ghrelin promotes cancer or inhibits its development and it is possible that it could have both stimulatory and inhibitory effects in different conditions. In most cell lines, ghrelin stimulates cell proliferation and is anti-apoptotic, apparently promoting cancer growth. On the contrary, in other models, cell proliferation is inhibited and apoptosis is favored. With such conflicting reports, further studies are required to establish the role of ghrelin in cancer cell growth and differentiation. If ghrelin had a pro-proliferative and anti-apoptotic action, ghrelin should probably be used with caution as a therapeutic agent to stimulate growth hormone release or for the treatment of cancer cachexia. Conversely, the inhibitory role on cell growth may be a valid therapeutic strategy to control tumor cell proliferation. Preventing the release of ghrelin into plasma through the use of specific blockers (e.g. octreotide) but providing cancerous tissue with local administration of exogenous ghrelin, as a growth factor antagonist, might be one of the possible applications in this direction. The clinical implications of this hypothesis, however, remain to be tested.

Ghrelin in Cancer Cell Proliferation

By now, several groups have documented that ghrelin promotes proliferation in a wide range of cancer cell lines, while others studies are in favor of an antiproliferative effect. An increase in proliferation has been found in cell line models from hematologic and solid cancers, including those from the adrenal cortex, prostate, breast, endometrium, pancreas, colorectum, and choriocarcinoma [33]. In most of them, such as prostate cancer cells, ghrelin-induced proliferation was mediated by the ERK1/2 MAPK pathway [18]. On the contrary, ghrelin inhibits or had no effect on proliferation in other models of thyroid [14], prostate [34, 35], breast [36] and small cell lung [8] carcinoma cell lines. Differences in ghrelin concentrations and methods for the evaluation of cell proliferation might be partially responsible for such controversial data – even in the same cellular model. Moreover, different clones of the same cell line might have heterogeneous phenotypes including ghrelin receptor expression, thus possibly changing the sensitivity and response to biological effects of ghrelin. Data from lung cancer cells clearly show that the pattern of ghrelin receptor expression is crucial for the proliferative response to ghrelin. In fact, ghrelin inhibited cell proliferation in the H345 small cell lung cancer cell line but not in Calu-1 squamous cell carcinoma cells that were inhibited by alternative synthetic peptide analogues of ghrelin (hexarelin and EP-80317), thus proving the existence of alternative ghrelin receptors [8, 9]. As further evidence, the effects on cell proliferation are also exerted by desacyl-ghrelin that is not capable of binding and activating GHSR 1a at physiological doses.

Ghrelin in Cancer Cell Apoptosis

As described above for proliferation, the role of ghrelin in regulating cancer cell apoptosis is not clear. Indeed, both proapoptotic and antiapoptotic effects have been demonstrated. A protective effect to chemotherapy-induced apoptosis has been demonstrated in endometrial [22] and colon [37] cancer cell models, and a baseline reduction of up to 20% apoptotic cells after ghrelin treatment was observed in SW-13 adrenocortical carcinoma cell line [38]. However, similar to that previously described for the ghrelin effects on cell proliferation (and possibly as the result of similar methodological and cell model variability), a marked increase in the basal apoptotic rate has been reported in SW-13 and H295R adrenocortical carcinoma [39], H345 small cell lung carcinoma [8] and PC3 prostate carcinoma [34] cell lines. Moreover, in esophageal carcinoma cells treated with a number of apoptosis-inducing agents, no specific effect of ghrelin on apoptosis was observed [40].

Ghrelin in Cancer Cells Migration and Invasion

Concerning cell motility and invasion there are only reports in favor of an inductor role of ghrelin. In particular, data on astrocytoma cell lines showed that ghrelin treatment increases cell migration in scratch assays and transwell assays and stimulates cell invasion in a dose-dependent manner [41] through the activation of the PI3K/Akt pathway [42]. Indeed, Waseem et al. [24] found that in colorectal cell lines, autocrine effects of ghrelin appear to stimulate cell invasion and migration, and these processes can be almost abolished in assays where cells are treated with the ghrelin antagonist, D(Lys-3)-GHRP-6, or by a ghrelin-neutralizing antibody.

Role of Obestatin in Cancer Growth Control and Progression

The biological effects of obestatin in neoplastic cell models are poorly understood. Our group investigated the role of obestatin in two human neuroendocrine cancer cell lines, derived from a medullary thyroid carcinoma (TT) and from a pancreatic neuroendocrine tumor (BON-1), both secreting obestatin at baseline [30]. The competition of endogenously secreted hormone with antiobestatin antibody had no effect on tumor cell proliferation and apoptosis, thus demonstrating the lack of an autocrine effect on cell growth by endogenous obestatin peptide in such cell models. In contrast, at pharmacological concentrations (up to 100 nM), obestatin demonstrated a negative effect on tumor cell proliferation in both TT and BON-1 cell lines, reaching statistical significance in the former. This effect was opposed to that of des-acylated ghrelin, which in both cell lines enhanced tumor growth, especially at higher doses [30].

Conclusion

From their original discovery in specific neuroendocrine cell types, ghrelin and obestatin were also identified in several tumors of neuroendocrine and nonneuroendocrine origin using different methods of investigation, being obestatin generally expressed in a subpopulation of ghrelin-positive tumor cells. In vitro studies on the capability of ghrelin (and, to a lower extent, obestatin) to modulate tumor cell function demonstrated an effect on the regulation of cell proliferation, apoptosis and invasiveness, although with variable and even paradoxical effects in different cell models. Although several methodological issues are possibly responsible for the controversial literature data, taken together all in vitro data suggest that ghrelin exerts different effects at physiological or pharmacological concentrations and that most of the pro- or antineoplastic properties are mediated by receptors alternative to GHSR1a, that still need to be identified. Therefore, the possible usefulness of the modulation of the ghrelin/obestatin axis in neoplastic conditions using either synthetic agonists or antagonists, though interesting in perspective, is still far from clinical applicability, and probably more related to the regulation of specific metabolic pathways in tumor cells, including lipid and carbohydrate use, than to a specific interference with cell proliferation.

References

1 Kojima M, Hosoda H, Date Y, Nakazato M, Matsuo H, Kangawa K: Ghrelin is a growth-hormone-releasing acylated peptide from stomach. Nature 1999;402:656–660.

2 Vu JP, Wang HS, Germano PM, Pisegna JR: Ghrelin in neuroendocrine tumors. Peptides 2011;32:2340–2347.

3 Rindi G, Savio A, Torsello A, Zoli M, Locatelli V, Cocchi D, Paolotti D, Solcia E: Ghrelin expression in gut endocrine growths. Histochem Cell Biol 2002;117:521–525.

4 Volante M, Allia E, Gugliotta P, Funaro A, Broglio F, Deghenghi R, Muccioli G, Ghigo E, Papotti M: Expression of ghrelin and of the GH secretagogue receptor by pancreatic islet cells and related endocrine tumors. J Clin Endocrinol Metab 2002;87:1300–1308.

5 Ekeblad S, Lejonklou MH, Grimfjard P, Johansson T, Eriksson B, Grimelius L, Stridsberg M, Stalberg P, Skogseid B: Co-expression of ghrelin and its receptor in pancreatic endocrine tumours. Clin Endocrinol (Oxf) 2007;66:115–122.

6 Korbonits M, Bustin SA, Kojima M, Jordan S, Adams EF, Lowe DG, Kangawa K, Grossman AB: The expression of the growth hormone secretagogue receptor ligand ghrelin in normal and abnormal human pituitary and other neuroendocrine tumors. J Clin Endocrinol Metab 2001;86:881–887.

7 Papotti M, Cassoni P, Volante M, Deghenghi R, Muccioli G, Ghigo E: Ghrelin-producing endocrine tumors of the stomach and intestine. J Clin Endocrinol Metab 2001;86:5052–5059.

8 Cassoni P, Allia E, Marrocco T, Ghe C, Ghigo E, Muccioli G, Papotti M: Ghrelin and cortistatin in lung cancer: expression of peptides and related receptors in human primary tumors and in vitro effect on the H345 small cell carcinoma cell line. J Endocrinol Invest 2006;29:781–790.

9 Ghe C, Cassoni P, Catapano F, Marrocco T, Deghenghi R, Ghigo E, Muccioli G, Papotti M: The antiproliferative effect of synthetic peptidyl GH secretagogues in human CALU-1 lung carcinoma cells. Endocrinology 2002;143:484–491.

10 Leontiou CA, Franchi G, Korbonits M: Ghrelin in neuroendocrine organs and tumours. Pituitary 2007;10:213–225.

11 Kim K, Arai K, Sanno N, Osamura RY, Teramoto A, Shibasaki T: Ghrelin and growth hormone (GH) secretagogue receptor (GHSR) mRNA expression in human pituitary adenomas. Clin Endocrinol (Oxf) 2001;54:759–768.

12 Kanamoto N, Akamizu T, Hosoda H, Hataya Y, Ariyasu H, Takaya K, Hosoda K, Saijo M, Moriyama K, Shimatsu A, Kojima M, Kangawa K, Nakao K: Substantial production of ghrelin by a human medullary thyroid carcinoma cell line. J Clin Endocrinol Metab 2001;86:4984–4990.

13 Morpurgo PS, Cappiello V, Verga U, Vicentini L, Vaghi I, Lauri E, Nebuloni M, Beck-Peccoz P, Spada A: Ghrelin in human medullary thyroid carcinomas. Clin Endocrinol (Oxf) 2005;63:437–441.

14 Volante M, Allia E, Fulcheri E, Cassoni P, Ghigo E, Muccioli G, Papotti M: Ghrelin in fetal thyroid and follicular tumors and cell lines: expression and effects on tumor growth. Am J Pathol 2003;162:645–654.

15 Cassoni P, Papotti M, Catapano F, Ghe C, Deghenghi R, Ghigo E, Muccioli G: Specific binding sites for synthetic growth hormone secretagogues in non-tumoral and neoplastic human thyroid tissue. J Endocrinol 2000;165:139–146.

16 Barzon L, Pacenti M, Masi G, Stefani AL, Fincati K, Palu G: Loss of growth hormone secretagogue receptor 1a and overexpression of type 1b receptor transcripts in human adrenocortical tumors. Oncology 2005;68:414–421.

17 Gaytan F, Barreiro ML, Caminos JE, Chopin LK, Herington AC, Morales C, Pinilla L, Paniagua R, Nistal M, Casanueva FF, Aguilar E, Dieguez C, Tena-Sempere M: Expression of ghrelin and its functional receptor, the type 1a growth hormone secretagogue receptor, in normal human testis and testicular tumors. J Clin Endocrinol Metab 2004;89:400–409.
18 Yeh AH, Jeffery PL, Duncan RP, Herington AC, Chopin LK: Ghrelin and a novel preproghrelin isoform are highly expressed in prostate cancer and ghrelin activates mitogen-activated protein kinase in prostate cancer. Clin Cancer Res 2005;11:8295–8303.
19 Grönberg M, Fjällskog ML, Jirström K, Janson ET: Expression of ghrelin is correlated to a favorable outcome in invasive breast cancer. Acta Oncol 2012;51: 386-393.
20 Jeffery PL, Murray RE, Yeh AH, McNamara JF, Duncan RP, Francis GD, Herington AC, Chopin LK: Expression and function of the ghrelin axis, including a novel preproghrelin isoform, in human breast cancer tissues and cell lines. Endocr Relat Cancer 2005; 12:839–850.
21 Gahete MD, Cordoba-Chacon J, Hergueta-Redondo M, Martinez-Fuentes AJ, Kineman RD, Moreno-Bueno G, Luque RM, Castano JP: A novel human ghrelin variant (In1-ghrelin) and ghrelin-O-acyltransferase are overexpressed in breast cancer: potential pathophysiological relevance. PLoS One 2011; 6:e23302.
22 Fung JN, Seim I, Wang D, Obermair A, Chopin LK, Chen C: Expression and in vitro functions of the ghrelin axis in endometrial cancer. Horm Cancer 2010;1: 245–255.
23 Dagli AF, Aydin S, Kocdor H, Gurates B, Sahin I, Catak Z, Ozercan MR, Ozercan IH: Ghrelin expression of endometrium hyperplasia and endometrioid carcinoma. Gynecol Endocrinol 2011;27:199–204.
24 Waseem T, Javaid Ur R, Ahmad F, Azam M, Qureshi MA: Role of ghrelin axis in colorectal cancer: a novel association. Peptides 2008;29:1369–1376.
25 Campa D, Pardini B, Naccarati A, Vodickova L, Novotny J, Steinke V, Rahner N, Holinski-Feder E, Morak M, Schackert HK, Gorgens H, Kotting J, Betz B, Kloor M, Engel C, Buttner R, Propping P, Forsti A, Hemminki K, Barale R, Vodicka P, Canzian F: Polymorphisms of genes coding for ghrelin and its receptor in relation to colorectal cancer risk: a two-step gene-wide case-control study. BMC Gastroenterol 2010;10:112.
26 Mottershead M, Karteris E, Barclay JY, Suortamo S, Newbold M, Randeva H, Nwokolo CU: Immunohistochemical and quantitative mRNA assessment of ghrelin expression in gastric and oesophageal adenocarcinoma. J Clin Pathol 2007;60:405–409.
27 Ekeblad S, Nilsson B, Lejonklou MH, Johansson T, Stalberg P, Nilsson O, Ahlman H, Skogseid B: Gastrointestinal stromal tumors express the orexigen ghrelin. Endocr Relat Cancer 2006;13:963–970.
28 Dagli AF, Aydin S, Karaoglu A, Akpolat N, Ozercan IH, Ozercan MR: Ghrelin expression in normal kidney tissue and renal carcinomas. Pathol Res Pract 2009;205:165–173.
29 Gaytan F, Morales C, Barreiro ML, Jeffery P, Chopin LK, Herington AC, Casanueva FF, Aguilar E, Dieguez C, Tena-Sempere M: Expression of growth hormone secretagogue receptor type 1a, the functional ghrelin receptor, in human ovarian surface epithelium, mullerian duct derivatives, and ovarian tumors. J Clin Endocrinol Metab 2005;90:1798–1804.
30 Volante M, Rosas R, Ceppi P, Rapa I, Cassoni P, Wiedenmann B, Settanni F, Granata R, Papotti M: Obestatin in human neuroendocrine tissues and tumours: expression and effect on tumour growth. J Pathol 2009;218:458–466.
31 Tsolakis AV, Grimelius L, Stridsberg M, Falkmer SE, Waldum HL, Saras J, Janson ET: Obestatin/ghrelin cells in normal mucosa and endocrine tumours of the stomach. Eur J Endocrinol 2009;160:941–949.
32 Karaoglu A, Aydin S, Dagli AF, Cummings DE, Ozercan IH, Canatan H, Ozkan Y: Expression of obestatin and ghrelin in papillary thyroid carcinoma. Mol Cell Biochem 2009;323:113–118.
33 Chopin L, Walpole C, Seim I, Cunningham P, Murray R, Whiteside E, Josh P, Herington A: Ghrelin and cancer. Mol Cell Endocrinol 2011;340:65–69.
34 Diaz-Lezama N, Hernandez-Elvira M, Sandoval A, Monroy A, Felix R, Monjaraz E: Ghrelin inhibits proliferation and increases T-type Ca^{2+} channel expression in PC-3 human prostate carcinoma cells. Biochem Biophys Res Commun 2010;403:24–29.
35 Cassoni P, Ghe C, Marrocco T, Tarabra E, Allia E, Catapano F, Deghenghi R, Ghigo E, Papotti M, Muccioli G: Expression of ghrelin and biological activity of specific receptors for ghrelin and des-acyl ghrelin in human prostate neoplasms and related cell lines. Eur J Endocrinol 2004;150:173–184.
36 Cassoni P, Papotti M, Ghe C, Catapano F, Sapino A, Graziani A, Deghenghi R, Reissmann T, Ghigo E, Muccioli G: Identification, characterization, and biological activity of specific receptors for natural (ghrelin) and synthetic growth hormone secretagogues and analogs in human breast carcinomas and cell lines. J Clin Endocrinol Metab 2001;86:1738–1745.
37 He XT, Fan XM, Zha XL: Ghrelin inhibits 5-fluorouracil-induced apoptosis in colonic cancer cells. J Gastroenterol Hepatol 2011;26:1169–1173.

38 Delhanty PJ, van Koetsveld PM, Gauna C, van de Zande B, Vitale G, Hofland LJ, van der Lely AJ: Ghrelin and its unacylated isoform stimulate the growth of adrenocortical tumor cells via an anti-apoptotic pathway. Am J Physiol Endocrinol Metab 2007;293:E302–E309.
39 Belloni AS, Macchi C, Rebuffat P, Conconi MT, Malendowicz LK, Parnigotto PP, Nussdorfer GG: Effect of ghrelin on the apoptotic deletion rate of different types of cells cultured in vitro. Int J Mol Med 2004;14:165–167.
40 Konturek PC, Burnat G, Rau T, Hahn EG, Konturek S: Effect of adiponectin and ghrelin on apoptosis of Barrett adenocarcinoma cell line. Dig Dis Sci 2008; 53:597–605.
41 Dixit VD, Weeraratna AT, Yang H, Bertak D, Cooper-Jenkins A, Riggins GJ, Eberhart CG, Taub DD: Ghrelin and the growth hormone secretagogue receptor constitute a novel autocrine pathway in astrocytoma motility. J Biol Chem 2006;281:16681–16690.
42 Duxbury MS, Waseem T, Ito H, Robinson MK, Zinner MJ, Ashley SW, Whang EE: Ghrelin promotes pancreatic adenocarcinoma cellular proliferation and invasiveness. Biochem Biophys Res Commun 2003;309:464–468.

Prof. Mauro Papotti
Department of Clinical and Biological Sciences, University of Turin, San Luigi Hospital
Regione Gonzole 10
IT–10043 Orbassano, Turin (Italy)
E-Mail mauro.papotti@unito.it

Benso A, Casanueva FF, Ghigo E, Granata A (eds): The Ghrelin System.
Endocr Dev. Basel, Karger, 2013, vol 25, pp 135–143 (DOI: 10.1159/000346064)

Ghrelin Function in Insulin Release and Glucose Metabolism

Katsuya Dezaki

Division of Integrative Physiology, Department of Physiology, Jichi Medical University School of Medicine, Shimotsuke, Japan

Abstract

Given its wide spectrum of biological activities such as growth hormone (GH) release, feeding stimulation, adiposity and cardiovascular actions, the discovery of ghrelin opened many new perspectives within neuroendocrine, metabolic and cardiovascular research, thus suggesting its possible clinical application. Circulating ghrelin is produced predominantly in the stomach, and its receptor GH secretagogue receptor (GHS-R) is expressed in a variety of central and peripheral tissues. Ghrelin, GHS-R and ghrelin *O*-acyltransferase (GOAT), the enzyme that promotes the acylation of the third serine residue of ghrelin, are all expressed in pancreatic islets, and this peptide is released into pancreatic microcirculations. Ghrelin inhibits insulin release in mice, rats and humans. The signal transduction mechanisms of ghrelin receptor in islet β-cells are very unique, being distinct from those utilized for GH release. Pharmacological and genetic blockade of islet-derived ghrelin markedly augments glucose-induced insulin release in vitro. Ablation of ghrelin, GHS-R or GOAT enhances insulin release and prevents impaired glucose tolerance in high-fat, diet-induced and leptin-deficient obese models. Thus, manipulation of the insulinostatic function of the ghrelin–GHS-R system, particularly that in islets, could optimize the amount of insulin release to meet the systemic demand. Ghrelin antagonism provides a novel strategy to treat type 2 diabetes with dysregulated insulin release.

Ghrelin, a stomach-derived 28-amino acid hormone discovered as the endogenous ligand for the growth hormone (GH) secretagogue receptor (GHS-R), potently stimulates GH release [1] and feeding [2] as well as exhibits adiposity [3] and positive cardiovascular effects [4]. Given this wide spectrum of biological activities, the discovery of ghrelin opened many new perspectives within neuroendocrine, metabolic and cardiovascular research, thus suggesting its possible clinical application. Recent evidence highlights an important role of ghrelin in glucose homeostasis. Ghrelin and GHS-R are also located in pancreatic islets [5, 6]. Ghrelin *O*-acyltransferase (GOAT), which has been identified as the enzyme that promotes the acylation of the third serine residue of ghrelin, is highly expressed in the pancreatic islets [7]. The concentrations of plasma ghrelin in the pancreatic vein are significantly higher than those in the pancreatic artery in rats, indicating that ghrelin is released from pancreas [8]. Ghrelin inhibits insulin release in mice, rats and humans [9–11]. Here, we review the physiological role of ghrelin in the regulation of insulin release and glucose metabolism, and present a potential therapeutic avenue to manipulate ghrelin signaling and thereby counteract the progression of type 2 diabetes.

Systemic Effects of Ghrelin on Insulin Release and Glucose Metabolism

Systemic action of exogenous ghrelin to elevate blood glucose levels has been well documented in humans and rodents. When ghrelin was simultaneously injected into mice with glucose in glucose tolerance test (GTT), the insulin responses were markedly attenuated and the glucose responses were larger in comparison to the control without ghrelin [11]. It has recently been shown that in healthy humans ghrelin suppresses insulin secretion and elevates blood glucose in intravenous GTT [12]. Conversely, GTT performed in mice showed that insulin responses were markedly enhanced and increases in plasma glucose were markedly attenuated by simultaneous injection of GHS-R antagonist [D-Lys^3]-GHRP-6 [11]. In insulin tolerance tests, hypoglycemic effect of insulin was indistinguishable between the ghrelin-injected, GHS-R antagonist-injected and control mice [11]. Esler et al. [13] confirmed these results by reporting that oral administration of a small molecule GHS-R antagonist improved glucose tolerance in rats by stimulating insulin secretion, while eliciting no apparent effect on insulin sensitivity. Pretreatment of mice with the GOAT inhibitor also showed increased insulin response and a reduced blood glucose in GTT [14]. Knockout studies support the pivotal role of ghrelin in glucose homeostasis. Mice lacking ghrelin [8, 15] have improved glucose tolerance mainly due to increased glucose-induced insulin secretion. Possible additional effects of ghrelin on glucose disposal or insulin sensitivity [15–18] cannot be disregarded.

Ghrelin as a Potential Therapeutic Target for Type 2 Diabetes

Circulating plasma ghrelin levels decrease immediately after a meal [19]. The meal-induced decrease of ghrelin levels is impaired in type 2 diabetic subjects [20], suggesting that the impaired suppression of circulating ghrelin during the meal intake may partly account for the glucose intolerance as well as ongoing weight gain in type 2 diabetes. When wild-type and ghrelin-KO mice were fed a high-fat diet (HFD), both mouse lines developed moderate increases in body weight to a similar extent [8]. In an apparent controversy, it was reported that another line of ghrelin-KO mice were protected from a rapid weight gain during post-weaning exposure to HFD, which was associated with decreased adiposity, increased energy expenditure and increased locomotor activity as compared to wild-type mice [21]. HFD treatment significantly increased blood glucose levels in wild-type mice but not in ghrelin-KO mice [8]. HFD treatment increased plasma insulin levels in wild-type mice, and this increment was much greater in ghrelin-KO. This phenotype was even more prominent in GTT. Ghrelin-deficiency promotes insulin release and prevents glucose intolerance in an HFD-induced obese model [8]. Sun et al. [15] have reported that ablation of ghrelin in leptin-deficient ob/ob mice augmented insulin release and thereby markedly reduced hyperglycemia. Thus, the ghrelin blockade counteracts the obesity-associated glucose intolerance in both the life style-related and genetic obese models. As the underlying mechanism, we propose that lack of ghrelin and its insulinostatic activity increase the maximal capacity of glucose-induced insulin release and enable islets to secrete more insulin to meet an increased demand associated with obesity, thereby achieving normoglycemia.

Insulinostatic Function of Ghrelin

To examine the physiological roles of the pancreatic islet-produced ghrelin, insulin release from the perfused rat pancreas, an in vitro system that retains the intact circulation in pancreatic islets while excluding the influence of other organs, was employed. The glucose-induced insulin release was significantly enhanced by blockade of GHS-R with a GHS-R antagonist and by immunoneutralization of endogenous ghrelin with antighrelin antiserum [8]. Conversely, administration of exogenous ghrelin suppressed it [8, 22]. In isolated rat islets, GHS-R antagonists and antiserum against ghrelin markedly increased glucose-stimulated insulin release [11]. The glucose-induced insulin release from isolated islets of ghrelin-KO mice was significantly greater than that of wild-type mice, while basal insulin release was not altered. No difference was observed between KO and wild-type mice in insulin content per islet and mRNA expressions of insulin 1 and insulin 2 [8]. These findings indicate that the endogenous ghrelin suppresses glucose-induced insulin secretion within islets. Barnett et al. [14] reported that pretreatment of human islet cells with a peptide-based GOAT inhibitor promoted significant increase in insulin response to a glucose challenge. These results indicate that GOAT may catalyze acylation of ghrelin in islets and confirm the insulinostatic function of islet-derived acyl-ghrelin suppresses insulin response in human.

Ghrelin Signaling Mechanisms in Islet β-Cells

Insulinostatic effects of ghrelin were blunted in rats pretreated with pertussis toxin (PTX), a specific inhibitor of Gi and Go subtypes of trimeric GTP-binding proteins [23]. In perfused pancreas of PTX-treated rats, glucose-induced insulin release was

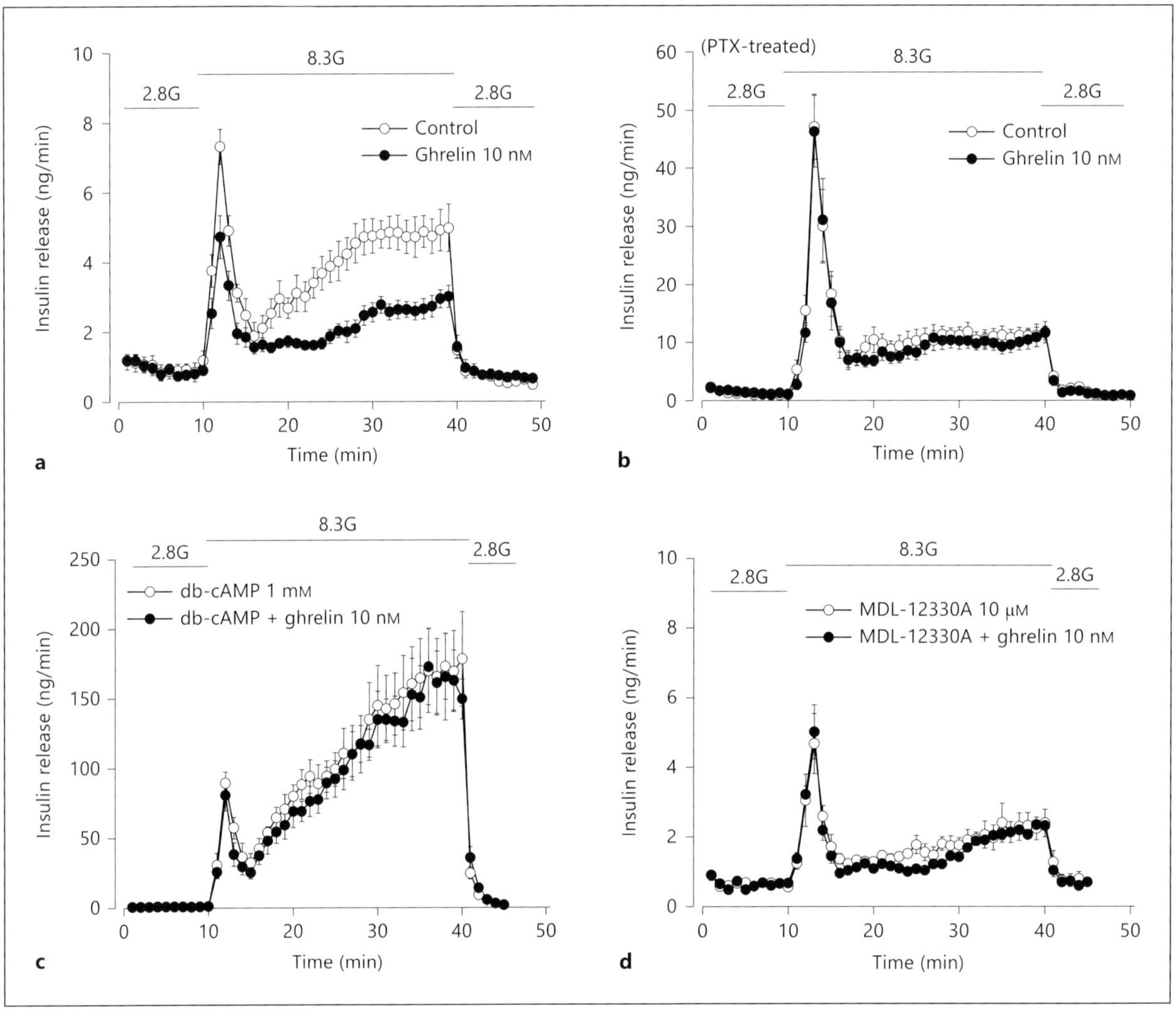

Fig. 1. Ghrelin suppresses 8.3 mM glucose (8.3G)-induced insulin release in perfused rat pancreas (**a**), but not in the perfused pancreas of PTX-treated rats (**b**). **c**, **d** In rat perfused pancreas, the insulinostatic ability of ghrelin is blunted when cellular cAMP level is clamped upward with a cAMP analogue dibutyryl-cAMP (db-cAMP) and downward with an adenylate cyclase inhibitor MDL-12330A. Copyright© 2011 American Diabetes Association from Dezaki et al. [25]. Reprinted with permission from The American Diabetes Association in a slightly modified form.

markedly enhanced, and ghrelin failed to affect it (fig. 1a, b). A membrane-permeable cAMP analogue, dibutyryl-cAMP (db-cAMP), markedly enhanced glucose-induced insulin release, and in the presence of db-cAMP, ghrelin failed to suppress the insulin release (fig. 1c). In the pancreas preincubated with an irreversible adenylate cyclase inhibitor, MDL-12330A, the glucose-induced insulin release was attenuated, and was not further altered by administration of ghrelin (fig. 1d). These results suggest that

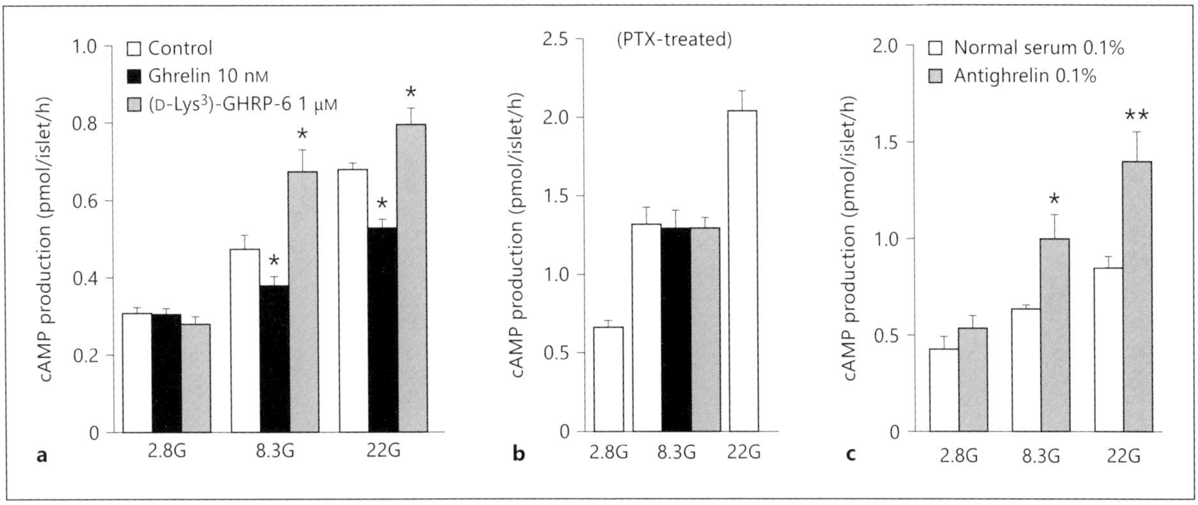

Fig. 2. a Glucose at 8.3 (8.3G) and 22 mM (22G) induces cAMP production in islets in the presence of phosphodiesterase inhibitor IBMX (500 μM). Exogenous ghrelin inhibits glucose-induced cAMP production, while a GHS-R antagonist [D-Lys^3]-GHRP-6 enhances it. **b** Neither ghrelin nor [D-Lys^3]-GHRP-6 alter glucose (8.3 mM)-induced cAMP production in islets isolated from PTX-treated rats. **c** Immunoneutralization of endogenous ghrelin with an antighrelin antiserum significantly enhances glucose-induced cAMP production.* $p < 0.05$, ** $p < 0.01$. Copyright© 2011 American Diabetes Association from Dezaki et al. [25]. Reprinted with permission from The American Diabetes Association in a slightly modified form.

ghrelin attenuates glucose-induced insulin release via the PTX-sensitive G- protein that is coupled to modulation of cAMP signaling. The glucose (8.3 and 22 mM)-induced cAMP production in isolated rat islets were significantly inhibited by exogenous ghrelin and augmented by GHS-R antagonist and antighrelin antiserum (fig. 2). Administration of ghrelin also suppressed the glucose-induced oscillatory rise in cytosolic cAMP concentrations in MIN6 β-cells transfected with a fluorescent-translocation biosensor using evanescent-wave microscopy, indicating that ghrelin directly inhibits glucose-induced cAMP signaling in β-cells [23].

At substimulatory glucose concentrations, β-cells maintain the resting membrane potential at a hyperpolarized level of around –70 mV. Elevation of the blood glucose concentration increases glucose uptake and metabolism by β-cells, resulting in closure of the ATP-sensitive K^+ (K_{ATP}) channels. When K^+ efflux is reduced, inward currents more effectively contribute to the membrane potential and depolarize the membrane, inducing bursting spike-like short action potentials at membrane potentials positive from –50 to –40 mV. These action potentials are produced by orchestrated openings of voltage-dependent Ca^{2+} channels and voltage-gated K^+ channels. The electrical firings were characterized by spike-like and repetitively occurring action potentials on top of the plateau phase of slow waves, and these firings were attenuated by ghrelin in a reversible manner [24]. In a study using patch clamp analysis, ghrelin increased the current amplitudes of the delayed rectifier K^+ (Kv) channel, but not the K_{ATP} and L-type Ca^{2+} channel ones, in rat single β-cells in a reversible manner. Ghrelin did not potentiate the Kv currents in the presence of membrane-permeable cyclic AMP analogues [11, 23, 24].

In rat single β-cells, ghrelin markedly suppressed the peak of the cytosolic Ca^{2+} concentration ($[Ca^{2+}]_i$) responses to 8.3 mM glucose and this effect was blocked by the GHS-R antagonist [11, 24]. The effects of ghrelin on the $[Ca^{2+}]_i$ responses were abolished in β-cells following exposure to PTX, suggesting that certain subtype(s) of PTX-sensitive G proteins are crucial in the ghrelin signal transduction in β-cells. Treatment of cultured rat β-cells with antisense oligonucleotide specific for the $G\alpha_{i2}$ subunit of G proteins markedly decreased $G\alpha_{i2}$ subunit expression and knocked down the ability of ghrelin to attenuate $[Ca^{2+}]_i$ responses and insulin release to glucose [24]. The action of ghrelin to suppress glucose-induced $[Ca^{2+}]_i$ increases was blunted in the β-cells whose cAMP levels were clamped upward by a cAMP analogue and downward by an adenylate cyclase inhibitor [23]. These results suggest that $G\alpha_{i2}$-mediated cAMP signaling is crucial for the action of ghrelin to suppress glucose-induced $[Ca^{2+}]_i$ increase and insulin release.

It has been reported that GHS-R is coupled to $G_{q/11}$-phospholipase C signaling, leading to production of IP_3 and Ca^{2+} release from IP_3-sensitive stores [25], and that ghrelin activates the phospholipase-C pathway for stimulating GH release in pituitary somatotrophs [26]. In contrast, the mechanisms by which GHS-R activates PTX-sensitive G_i proteins and decreases cAMP in β-cells are unclear. G protein-coupled receptors often activate more than one type of G protein. Hence, the ghrelin interaction with GHS-R could activate distinct classes of G protein signaling in a tissue-specific manner. Alternatively, the isoforms of GHS-R or heterodimer of GHS-R with other receptors could access the G_i protein complex. The ghrelin receptor in β-cells remains to be further characterized.

Conclusion

Ghrelin, including that produced by pancreatic islets, plays a pivotal role in the regulation of insulin release and blood glucose in rodents and humans. Ghrelin attenuates the glucose-induced cAMP production, which drives activation of Kv channels and suppression of the glucose-induced $[Ca^{2+}]_i$ increase and insulin release in islet β-cells (fig. 3). This novel ghrelin signaling in β-cells is distinct from that reported in other tissues including pituitary GH cells. Ghrelin may elicit different signaling pathways in a tissue-specific manner, which may underlie the opposing effects of ghrelin on GH release and insulin release. When the systemic demand for insulin exceeds the physiological range, including insulin resistance and obesity, antagonism of ghrelin function can promote insulin secretion and thereby prevent glucose

Fig. 3. Ghrelin elicits different signaling pathways in a tissue-specific manner. In pituitary GH cells, GHS-R is coupled to $G_{q/11}$-phospholipase C (PLC) signaling, leading to production of IP_3 and diacylglycerol (DG), and Ca^{2+} release from IP_3-sensitive stores, and that ghrelin activates PLC pathway for stimulating GH release. In contrast, ghrelin attenuates the glucose-induced cAMP production via activation of the Gi-coupled receptor, which drives activation of Kv channels and suppression of the glucose-induced $[Ca^{2+}]_i$ increase and insulin release in islet β-cells.

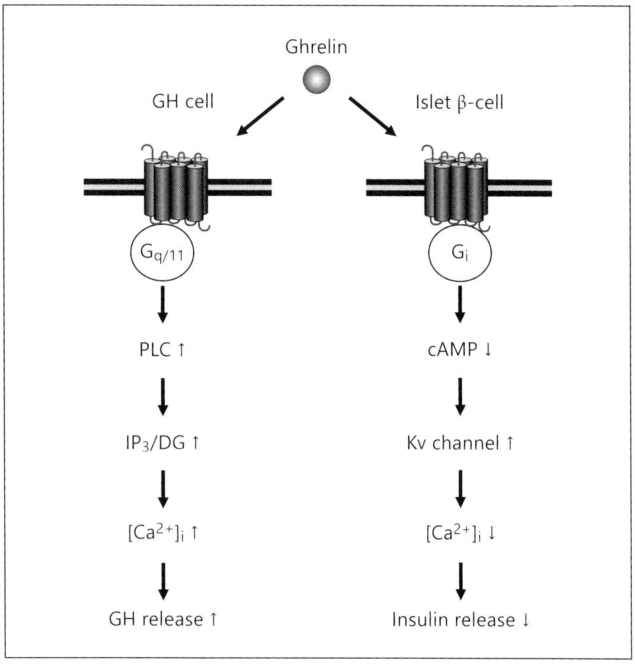

intolerance, providing a potential therapeutic avenue to counteract the progression of type 2 diabetes. As the cAMP pathway is the major signaling route of incretin hormones such as glucagon-like peptide 1 (GLP-1) in islet β-cells, interaction between ghrelin and GLP-1 plays an important role in physiological regulation of glucose-induced insulin release in islet β-cells, and blockade of endogenous ghrelin provides a novel tool to enhance therapeutic ability of GLP-1 and GLP-1-based drugs and to minimize the doses of these drugs and thereby to reduce the side effects. It is of particular importance to clarify how ghrelin and its receptor in islets are regulated under physiological and pathological conditions, including fast/fed, lean/obese and normoglycemic/diabetic states. Precise and relative roles of islet-derived vs. stomach-derived ghrelin in multiple steps of glucose metabolism remain to be further clarified.

Acknowledgments

This work was supported by grants-in-aid for Scientific Research and that on Priority Areas from the Japan Society for the Promotion of Science, by grants from the Salt Science Research Foundation, the Pharmacological Research Foundation, Tokyo and Takeda Science Foundation to K.D.

References

1 Kojima M, Hosoda H, Date Y, Nakazato M, Matsuo H, Kangawa K: Ghrelin is a growth-hormone-releasing peptide from stomach. Nature 1999;402:656–660.

2 Nakazato M, Murakami N, Date Y, Kojima M, Matsuo H, Kangawa K, Matsukura S: A role for ghrelin in the central regulation of feeding. Nature 2001;409:194–198.

3 Tschöp M, Smiley DL, Heiman ML: Ghrelin induces adiposity in rodents. Nature 2000;407:908–913.

4 Nagaya N, Kojima M, Uematsu M, Yamagishi M, Hosoda H, Oya H, Hayashi Y, Kangawa K: Hemodynamic and hormonal effects of human ghrelin in healthy volunteers. Am J Physiol 2001;280:R1483–R1487.

5 Date Y, Nakazato M, Hashiguchi S, Dezaki K, Mondal MS, Hosoda H, Kojima M, Kangawa K, Arima T, Matsuo H, Yada T, Matsukura S: Ghrelin is present in pancreatic α-cells of humans and rats and stimulates insulin secretion. Diabetes 2002;51:124–129.

6 Gnanapavan S, Kola B, Bustin SA, Morris DG, McGee P, Fairclough P, Bhattacharya S, Carpenter R, Grossman AB, Korbonits M: The tissue distribution of the mRNA of ghrelin and subtypes of its receptor, GHS-R, in humans. J Clin Endocrinol Metab 2002;87:2988–2991.

7 An W, Li Y, Xu G, Zhao J, Xiang X, Ding L, Li J, Guan Y, Wang X, Tang C, Li X, Mulholland M, Zhang W: Modulation of ghrelin O-acyltransferase expression in pancreatic islets. Cell Physiol Biochem 2010;26:707–716.

8 Dezaki K, Sone H, Koizumi M, Nakata M, Kakei M, Nagai H, Hosoda H, Kangawa K, Yada T: Blockade of pancreatic islet-derived ghrelin enhances insulin secretion to prevent high-fat diet-induced glucose intolerance. Diabetes 2006;55:3486–3493.

9 Broglio F, Arvat E, Benso A, Gottero C, Muccioli G, Papotti M, van der Lely AJ, Deghenghi R, Ghigo E: Ghrelin, a natural GH secretagogue produced by the stomach, induces hyperglycemia and reduces insulin secretion in humans. J Clin Endocrinol Metab 2001;86:5083–5086.

10 Reimer MK, Pacini G, Ahrén B: Dose-dependent inhibition by ghrelin of insulin secretion in the mouse. Endocrinology 2003;144:916–921.

11 Dezaki K, Hosoda H, Kakei M, Hashiguchi S, Watanabe M, Kangawa K, Yada T: Endogenous ghrelin in pancreatic islets restricts insulin release by attenuating Ca^{2+} signaling in β-cells: implication in the glycemic control in rodents. Diabetes 2004;53:3142–3151.

12 Tong J, Prigeon RL, Davis HW, Bidlingmaier M, Kahn SE, Cummings DE, Tschöp MH, D'Alessio D: Ghrelin suppresses glucose-stimulated insulin secretion and deteriorates glucose tolerance in healthy humans. Diabetes 2010;59:2145–2151.

13 Esler WP, Rudolph J, Claus TH, Tang W, Barucci N, Brown SE, Bullock W, Daly M, Decarr L, Li Y, Milardo L, Molstad D, Zhu J, Gardell SJ, Livingston JN, Sweet LJ: Small-molecule ghrelin receptor antagonists improve glucose tolerance, suppress appetite, and promote weight loss. Endocrinology 2007;148:5175–5185.

14 Barnett BP, Hwang Y, Taylor MS, Kirchner H, Pfluger PT, Bernard V, Lin YY, Bowers EM, Mukherjee C, Song WJ, Longo PA, Leahy DJ, Hussain MA, Tschöp MH, Boeke JD, Cole PA: Glucose and weight control in mice with a designed ghrelin O-acyltransferase inhibitor. Science 2010;330:1689–1692.

15 Sun Y, Asnicar M, Saha PK, Chan L, Smith RG: Ablation of ghrelin improves the diabetic but not obese phenotype of ob/ob mice. Cell Metab 2006;3:379–386.

16 Gauna C, Delhanty PJ, Hofland LJ, Janssen JA, Broglio F, Ross RJ, Ghigo E, van der Lely AJ: Ghrelin stimulates, whereas des-octanoyl ghrelin inhibits, glucose output by primary hepatocytes. J Clin Endocrinol Metab 2005;90:1055–1060.

17 Heijboer AC, van den Hoek AM, Parlevliet ET, Havekes LM, Romijn JA, Pijl H, Corssmit EP: Ghrelin differentially affects hepatic and peripheral insulin sensitivity in mice. Diabetologia 2006;49:732–738.

18 Longo KA, Govek EK, Nolan A, McDonagh T, Charoenthongtrakul S, Giuliana DJ, Morgan K, Hixon J, Zhou C, Kelder B, Kopchick JJ, Saunders JO, Navia MA, Curtis R, DiStefano PS, Geddes BJ: Pharmacologic inhibition of ghrelin receptor signaling is insulin sparing and promotes insulin sensitivity. J Pharmacol Exp Ther 2011;339:115–124.

19 Cummings DE, Purnell JQ, Frayo RS, Schmidova K, Wisse BE, Weigle DS: A preprandial rise in plasma ghrelin levels suggests a role in meal initiation in humans. Diabetes 2001;50:1714–1719.

20 Rudovich N, Möhlig M, Otto B, Pivovarova O, Spranger J, Weickert MO, Pfeiffer AF: Effect of meglitinides on postprandial ghrelin secretion pattern in type 2 diabetes mellitus. Diabetes Technol Ther 2010;12:57–64.

21 Wortley KE, del Rincon JP, Murray JD, Garcia K, Iida K, Thorner MO, Sleeman MW: Absence of ghrelin protects against early-onset obesity. J Clin Invest 2005;115:3573–3578.

22 Egido EM, Rodriguez-Gallardo J, Silvestre RA, Marco J: Inhibitory effect of ghrelin on insulin and pancreatic somatostatin secretion. Eur J Endocrinol 2002;146:241–244.
23 Dezaki K, Damdindorj B, Sone H, Dyachok O, Tengholm A, Gylfe E, Kurashina T, Yoshida M, Kakei M, Yada T: Ghrelin attenuates cAMP-PKA signaling to evoke insulinostatic cascade in islet β-cells. Diabetes 2011;60:2315–2324.
24 Dezaki K, Kakei M, Yada T: Ghrelin uses $G\alpha_{i2}$ and activates Kv channels to attenuate glucose-induced Ca^{2+} signaling and insulin release in islet β-cells: Novel signal transduction of ghrelin. Diabetes 2007; 56:2319–2327.
25 Howard AD, Feighner SD, Cully DF, et al: A receptor in pituitary and hypothalamus that functions in growth hormone release. Science 1996;273:974–977.
26 Malagón MM, Luque RM, Ruiz-Guerrero E, Rodríguez-Pacheco F, García-Navarro S, Casanueva FF, Gracia-Navarro F, Castaño JP: Intracellular signaling mechanisms mediating ghrelin-stimulated growth hormone release in somatotropes. Endocrinology 2003;144:5372–5380.

Katsuya Dezaki
Division of Integrative Physiology, Department of Physiology, Jichi Medical University School of Medicine
Yakushiji 3311–1
Shimotsuke, Tochigi 329-0498 (Japan)
E-Mail dezaki@jichi.ac.jp

Benso A, Casanueva FF, Ghigo E, Granata A (eds): The Ghrelin System.
Endocr Dev. Basel, Karger, 2013, vol 25, pp 144–156 (DOI: 10.1159/000346306)

Products of the Ghrelin Gene, the Pancreatic β-Cell and the Adipocyte

Riccarda Granata · Ezio Ghigo

Department of Medical Sciences, Division of Endocrinology, Diabetology and Metabolism, University of Turin, Turin, Italy

Abstract

The ghrelin system comprises acylated ghrelin (AG), unacylated ghrelin (UAG) and obestatin, besides the receptor for AG, the growth hormone (GH) secretagogue receptor type 1a (GHS-R1a), and the enzyme-promoting ghrelin acylation, ghrelin *O*-acyltransferase (GOAT). The ghrelin peptides exert a variety of biological actions, including regulation of energy homeostasis and glucose metabolism, as well as survival and proliferative effects in different cell types. Besides the stomach, its main site of production, ghrelin is expressed in pancreatic islets, where it represents an independent islet cell population. AG exerts insulinostatic actions, UAG has been shown to oppose the AG inhibitory effects on insulin secretion, and obestatin has demonstrated insulinotropic activities. Although differences exist in the regulation of glucose homeostasis, all peptides display survival and antiapoptotic actions in pancreatic β-cells, preserving β-cell mass and function both in vitro and in vivo. The ghrelin system is also expressed in adipose tissue, and ghrelin effects have been demonstrated in both white and brown adipocytes. Indeed, AG, UAG and obestatin promote adipogenesis and glucose uptake, and inhibit adipocyte lipolysis. Interestingly, despite similar effects at the cellular level, results from ghrelin, GHS-R and GOAT knockout mice have indicated that AG display diabetogenic effects in vivo. Conversely, UAG and obestatin positively regulate glucose metabolism, and a new role has been recently proposed for obestatin on adipocyte function and insulin sensitivity.

Ghrelin, a 28-amino acid peptide produced by the stomach, was discovered as endogenous ligand for the growth hormone (GH) secretagogue receptor type 1a (GHS-R1a) [1]. Ghrelin potently stimulates GH release and food intake, induces adiposity and exerts a wide range of central and peripheral actions [2]. Ghrelin acylation on the third serine residue, promoted by ghrelin *O*-acyltransferase (GOAT), is essential for binding to GHS-R1a and for the central activities of the peptide [3–5]. Besides the stomach, acylated ghrelin (AG) and GHS-R1a are produced in different central and peripheral tissues, including the pancreas and adipose tissue [6–10].

Ghrelin peptides exist in two major forms, acylated ghrelin (AG) and unacylated ghrelin (UAG), of which UAG is the most abundant [1, 11]. UAG, like AG, is mainly produced in the stomach; however, it is devoid of binding to GHS-R1a and therefore unable to stimulate GH release and food intake. Nonetheless, UAG exerts many biological activities, some of which similar and other opposed to or independent of AG. Interestingly, AG and UAG display the same effects in different cell types and recognize common binding sites, suggesting the existence of a yet unknown receptor which is bound by both peptides [12–15].

Obestatin was recently discovered as a 23-amino acid amidated peptide encoded by the ghrelin gene [16]. Initially identified as the ligand of the orphan receptor GPR39, obestatin was claimed to oppose ghrelin effects on food intake [16, 17]; however, both findings have been questioned and to date obestatin physiological role has yet to be defined [18, 19]. Like ghrelin, obestatin is produced in the gastrointestinal tract, as well as in central and peripheral tissues [20]. Moreover, it exerts both central and peripheral actions and has been recently found to play a role in pancreatic β-cell survival and function [21], as well as in adipocyte function and glucose metabolism [22–24].

The role of the ghrelin gene-derived peptides in the pancreas and adipose tissue is becoming an important topic, particularly in light of the potential therapeutic applications in conditions such as obesity and insulin resistance. The present review highlights the most recent findings on AG, UAG and obestatin functions in pancreatic β-cells and adipocytes; indeed, these cells play a major role in glucose and lipid metabolism (fig. 1).

Ghrelin System in the Endocrine Pancreas

Ghrelin and GHS-R1a expression have been demonstrated in both human and rodent pancreatic islets [6, 7, 12, 20, 25, 26] and ghrelin in fetal life was found to be more abundant in the pancreas than in the stomach, suggesting a paracrine/autocrine role of the ghrelin system in hormonal secretion and/or islet growth and differentiation [27, 28]. Interestingly, ghrelin-producing ε-cells have been identified in pancreatic islets, and during fetal development ε-cells showed an ontogenetic and morphogenetic pattern distinct from that of glucagon-producing α-cells and insulin-producing β-cells [28–30].

In the developing mouse and rat pancreas, ghrelin immunoreactivity can be detected as early as embryonic day E9.5 and E15, respectively, and remains positive throughout gestation, peaking just before birth [30, 31]. Notably, ε-cells replaced β-cells and most of α-cells in two mouse models of pancreas development, suggesting a relationship between ghrelin-, insulin- and glucagon-producing cells in the developing pancreas [31, 32]. In normal adult rats, ghrelin immunoreactivity has been observed in the peripheral region, whereas in diabetic rats, it was found in the central region of the islets [33].

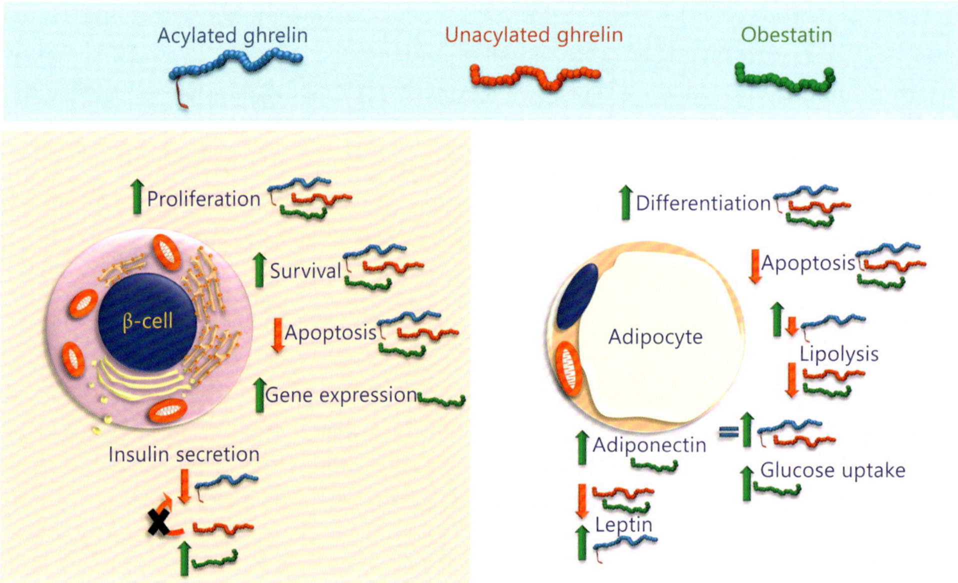

Fig. 1. Effects of the ghrelin gene-derived peptides in the pancreatic β-cell and the adipocyte. Acylated ghrelin (blue), unacylated ghrelin (red) and obestatin (green) exert both similar and opposed actions. Only the most important effects are indicated and in some cases, such as gene expression (regulation of genes involved in β-cell survival, differentiation and function, left panel), data are obtained from studies performed with only one of the three peptides.

In humans, ε-cells have been detected from midgestation to early postnatal period, accounting for approximately 10% of all islet cells [28, 29]. The developmental pattern of the ghrelin cells in human pancreas, although clearly distinct, was found to be quite similar to that of glucagon-expressing cells. Indeed, in fetal pancreas, ε- and α-cells reside at the periphery of the islets, whereas β-cells are mostly located in the islet core [26, 34–36]. Interestingly, colocalization of ghrelin and glucagon has been shown in both human and rat pancreas, which further supports the possible developmental link between these two cell types [6, 30]. Recently, ghrelin immunostaining was found to be either dependent or independent of glucagon, suggesting the existence of two different pancreatic ghrelin cell populations [37].

With regard to GHS-R1a, its immunoreactivity in human pancreatic islets partially overlaps with that of insulin in β-cells, in agreement with the many findings on β-cell responsiveness to ghrelin stimulation [12, 38]. Moreover, like ghrelin, GHS-R1a is expressed in human and rat developing pancreatic islets, from early gestation to adult [12, 27, 39].

Obestatin colocalizes with ghrelin at the periphery of the islets in rat, as well as in fetal and adult human pancreas [20, 21, 37, 40, 41]. Furthermore, both human pancreatic islets and INS-1E β-cells were found able to release obestatin, suggesting autocrine/paracrine effects of the peptide [21]. Besides the different ghrelin gene products, high levels of GOAT mRNA have been found in both stomach and pancreas [3], indicating regulatory mechanisms controlling AG versus UAG production and the consequent effects of these peptides on glucose metabolism and/or cell proliferation and survival.

Ghrelin Gene-Derived Peptides and the Pancreatic β-Cell

Different studies have shown that AG, UAG and obestatin play key roles in pancreatic β-cells and human pancreatic islets [38, 42]. We will not describe here their effects on insulin secretion and glucose metabolism, as they will be thoroughly covered in the chapter by Dezaki et al. [this vol.]. We will focus instead on β-cell proliferation and survival, and the underlying signaling pathways triggered by the peptides.

The survival and antiapoptotic effects of the ghrelin gene products have been described in a variety of cell types [43]. Interestingly, AG and UAG, when investigated together, showed similar ability to increase cell proliferation and survival and to inhibit apoptosis. Due to UAG inability to bind to GHSR-1a, it was proposed the existence of an alternative receptor involved in these effects [12, 13, 15, 44].

In HIT-T15 and INS-1E β-cells, as well as in human pancreatic islets, AG and UAG promote proliferation and inhibit apoptosis induced by serum starvation and cytokine synergism, which is a main cause of β-cell destruction in diabetes [12, 45, 46]. HIT-T15 cells do not express GHS-R1a, and possess common binding sites for AG and UAG, in agreement with previous studies which postulated the existence of a common receptor recognized by both peptides [15, 44, 47]. AG and UAG survival effects in β-cells involved signaling through the $G\alpha_s$ protein-coupled receptor and adenylyl cyclase (AC)/3′,5′-cyclic AMP (cAMP)/protein kinase A (PKA) pathway, and activation of survival and proliferative cascades such as phosphatidyl inositol-3 kinase (PI3K)/Akt and extracellular signal-regulated kinase (ERK)1/2. Autocrine or paracrine effects of AG and UAG were also suggested, due to their release in β-cell conditioned medium and to increased β-cell apoptosis after incubation with anti-ghrelin antibodies [12]. Both peptides even reduced cytokine-induced nitric oxide production, which is also a cause of β-cell dysfunction and death [48]. Other studies have later shown antiapoptotic effects of AG in HIT-T15 β-cells [49] and inhibitory effects against lipotoxicity-induced apoptosis in MIN6 β-cells, where AG activated protein kinase B (PKB), inhibited JNK signaling and nuclear translocation of forkhead box protein O1 (Foxo1) [50, 51].

On the basis of the greater positive effects on insulin sensitivity and glucose homeostasis, UAG was suggested to be a more appealing candidate for the treatment of metabolic dysfunctions, such as insulin resistance and type 2 diabetes. Therefore, studies were performed to assess whether UAG fragments would mimic the actions of full length peptide on survival of β-cells and human pancreatic islets. These fragments either included or excluded serine-3, the site for ghrelin acylation essential for binding to GHS-R. It was demonstrated that like their parent molecule, UAG fragments, particularly $UAG_{(6-13)}$, increase survival of β-cells and human pancreatic islets, prevent streptozotocin (STZ)-induced diabetes in rats, and reduce oxidative stress and senescence in human endothelial progenitor cells (EPCs) [52]. Therefore, UAG fragments may be promising therapeutic tools for preservation of β-cell mass and impaired vascular growth in metabolic dysfunctions and diabetes.

Like ghrelin, obestatin is secreted by β-cells and human islets of Langerhans and elicits proliferative and antiapoptotic effects in these cells through the cAMP pathway and activation of ERK1/2 and PI3K/Akt [21]. Interestingly, differently from AG, which has been mostly found to inhibit glucose-induced insulin secretion [38], obestatin promotes insulin secretion in vitro, in β-cell lines and human pancreatic islets [21], as well as in vivo [23] and in the perfused rat pancreas [53]. Notably, the glucagon-like peptide 1 receptor (GLP-1R) was found to be involved in obestatin actions in β-cells, as demonstrated by the inhibitory effect of the GLP-1R antagonist exendin-9 (Ex9) on obestatin-induced β-cell survival, by obestatin binding affinity for GLP-1R and by results showing the obestatin-induced increase of GLP-1R mRNA [21]. Moreover, like the GLP-1R agonist exendin-4 (Ex4), obestatin increases gene expression and phosphorylation of insulin receptor substrate-2 (IRS-2), which is implicated in both insulin receptor (IR) and GLP-1R signaling [21]. Due to the many evidence against GPR39 as the obestatin receptor [18, 54], these new findings are attractive and suggest that obestatin may at least partly signal through the GLP-1R.

In human islets, obestatin also promotes the phosphorylation of cAMP response element-binding protein (CREB) [21], which regulates glucose homeostasis and β-cell survival [55]. In addition, it decreases the phosphorylation of Src [21], whose expression in β-cells has been related to inhibition of Ca^{2+}-dependent insulin secretion [56]. Furthermore, in human islets obestatin upregulates gene expression of pancreatic and duodenal homeobox 1 (PDX-1), IRS-2, GLP-1R and glucokinase, which are key players in β-cell differentiation, survival and function. Notably, besides being produced by human pancreatic islets, obestatin expression has been demonstrated in both fetal and adult pancreas, colocalizing with ghrelin, likely in ε-cells, but not with the other islet hormones [20, 21, 40].

The survival effects of the ghrelin gene-derived peptides in the endocrine pancreas are not limited to β-cells. Indeed, a recent study has described the antiapoptotic action of AG, UAG and obestatin in human pancreatic islet microendothelial cells (MECs) exposed to chronic hyperglycemia [57]. These effects were similar to those of Ex4 and involved the same pathways as those of β-cells, suggesting that the peptides may improve islet vascularization and, indirectly, islet cell function.

In vivo, AG was found to promote β-cell regeneration and to increase insulin expression and secretion in newborn rats treated with STZ [58], a compound traditionally used to study pancreatic regeneration which specifically induces β-cell destruction [59]. Similar effects were recently demonstrated with UAG and obestatin. Indeed, in the pancreas of STZ-treated rats UAG and obestatin reduced glucose levels, promoted insulin expression and secretion, as well as PDX-1 mRNA. Furthermore, they increased pancreatic islet area and number, and expression of the antiapoptotic Bcl-2 protein [58]. Both AG and obestatin have also been shown to inhibit the development of acute pancreatitis, as demonstrated by an improvement of pancreatic histology and a decrease in biochemical indexes of the severity of acute pancreatitis. In addition, they decreased serum concentration of the proinflammatory cytokine IL-1β, suggesting that besides the survival effects in β-cells they reduce inflammation [60, 61]. In pancreatectomized rats, which are hyperglycemic and have reduced β-cell mass and insulin levels, AG was found to improve glycemia and increase insulin levels and insulin-positive islet cell number. Conversely, ghrelin receptor antagonists increased glucose levels and decreased the number of β-cells, suggesting the involvement of endogenous AG in islet cell survival and function [62].

Ghrelin Gene-Derived Peptides and Adipocytes

White adipose tissue (WAT) plays a key role in regulating energy homeostasis and endocrine functions, through the secretion of hormones and adipokines influencing pathophysiological events such as growth and differentiation, glucose homeostasis, obesity and cancer [63].

Expression of the ghrelin gene products, both at the mRNA and protein level, has been demonstrated in human and rodent adipocytes [1, 9, 10, 23, 24, 64, 65]. Similarly, GHS-R1a is expressed in adipocytes and in rodent and human adipose tissue [10, 22, 24, 64–70], although opposite findings have also been shown [8, 47, 71]. AG and UAG also bind to common receptor(s) in adipocytes, suggesting the existence of a yet unknown receptor, likely different from GHS-R1a [47].

In vivo, both intracerebroventricular and intraperitoneal administration of AG in rodents induces adiposity [72, 73] and promotes the increase of fat storage-promoting enzymes in WAT [74]. Also UAG, like AG, has been shown to promote adiposity in vivo and the effects of both peptides were found to be either independent of GHS-R1a [75] or of the AG orexigenic effect [69, 76]. Interestingly, mice overexpressing UAG in adipose tissue showed reduced fat mass and resistance to high fat diet-induced obesity; moreover, these mice demonstrated improved insulin sensitivity and glucose tolerance, suggesting positive effects of UAG in glucose metabolism [77]. Furthermore, in GHS-R deleted mice UAG suppressed the expression of genes involved in lipid metabolism, particularly those related to lipogenesis, in WAT and muscle, suggesting direct, GHSR-independent action of UAG to improve insulin sensitivity and metabolic profile [78].

AG adipogenic action was also observed in brown adipose tissue (BAT), where the peptide either decreased or increased the expression of uncoupling protein (UCP) mRNA [74, 79]. Another study failed to demonstrate any effect of AG on BAT accumulation, although increased mitogen-activated protein kinase activity and decreased adiponectin gene expression was observed [80]. In rats, both intracerebroventricular and intraperitoneal administration of AG reduced noradrenaline release in BAT, suggesting an important role of AG in the regulation of energy metabolism through suppression of the sympathetic nervous system innervating brown adipocytes [81]. AG has been also found to promote leptin secretion from rat white adipocytes [82], whereas UAG exhibited opposite effects in human adipocytes [9]. GHS-R ablation in aging mice was recently shown to reduce glucose/lipid uptake and lipogenesis in WAT and to increase thermogenic capacity in BAT, suggesting that GHS-R may be an important regulator of lipid metabolism during normal aging [83].

In agreement with most in vivo data, different studies have reported ghrelin-induced adipocyte differentiation in vitro [10, 22, 65, 66]. In 3T3-L1 preadipocytes, AG promotes cell proliferation and glucose uptake, inhibits apoptosis, activates PI3K/Akt and ERK1/2 signaling and induces adipocyte differentiation [65]. Conversely, ghrelin overexpression in 3T3-L1 adipocytes and AG administration to these cells was also reported to reduce adipocyte differentiation, through increased cell proliferation and mitogen-activated protein kinase activity, and inhibition of peroxisome proliferator-activator receptor-γ (PPAR-γ) [71].

Both AG and UAG exert antilipolytic activity in vitro in rat adipocytes [22, 47, 66, 84]. These effects were recently found to involve PI3Kγ/Akt and phosphodiesterase (PDE) and signaling through a common receptor bound by both peptides [84]. In human adipocytes isolated from subcutaneous abdominal fat UAG, but not AG, showed inhibition of lipolysis [9]. Accordingly, recent data indicated that UAG improves glucose metabolism and reduces lipolysis in vivo in healthy volunteers [14]. Furthermore, AG infusion in humans acutely induced lipolysis and insulin resistance, independently of GH and cortisol secretion [85].

Different studies have also demonstrated AG and UAG effects on glucose and fatty acid uptake. AG and UAG either stimulate or have no effect on glucose uptake in 3T3-L1 adipocytes [9, 22, 65, 67]. AG and UAG have been also found to increase fatty acid uptake in 3T3-L1 adipocyte, and AG infusion promoted hepatic steatosis in rats via a GHS-R1a-dependent mechanism [68].

Recently, obestatin effects have been demonstrated in adipocytes, both in vitro and in vivo. These studies suggested that obestatin plays a positive role on adipocyte function and glucose metabolism [22–24]. Obestatin stimulates proliferation and inhibits apoptosis in 3T3-L1 adipocytes, and its antiapoptotic effect involves activation of PI3K/Akt and ERK1/2 signaling [22, 23]. Obestatin promotes the differentiation of both 3T3-L1 and human subcutaneous (SC)- and omental (OM)-derived adipocytes, and increases the expression of adipogenic genes [22–24]. Furthermore, it inhibits lipolysis in 3T3-L1 cells [22, 23] and human SC and OM adipocytes isolated from both lean and obese individuals [23]. Similar inhibitory actions were observed for non-esterified fatty acid (NEFA) release in 3T3-L1 cells [22].

Activation of AMP-activated protein kinase (AMPK) has been shown to antagonize lipolysis in adipocytes, and obestatin was found to either promote AMPK phosphorylation in 3T3-L1 and human SC adipocytes [23] or to inactivate AMPK in 3T3-L1 [24]. Furthermore, in human SC adipocytes, obestatin, used in the nanomolar range, increased adiponectin and reduced leptin secretion [23]. Moreover, it promoted glucose uptake in both 3T3-L1 [23, 24] and human SC adipocytes, as well as translocation of the glucose transporter GLUT4 [23]. Sirtuin 1 (SIRT1), which has been reported to increase glucose transport and insulin signaling in adipocytes [86], was increased by obestatin and involved in obestatin stimulatory effect on glucose uptake, as demonstrated by studies using small interfering RNA (siRNA) [23]. Obestatin also increased PI3K/Akt phosphorylation in 3T3-L1 and human SC adipocytes, as well as the Akt downstream pathways GSK-3β, mTOR and S6K1. Moreover, Akt activation was demonstrated in vivo in WAT of rats infused with obestatin [23, 24]. Obestatin also potently increased free fatty acid uptake in 3T3-L1 adipocytes [22]. Interestingly, obestatin showed binding specificity for both 3T3-L1 and human SC preadipocytes and differentiated adipocytes, which was displaced by both the GLP-1R agonist exendin-4 (Ex-4) and the antagonist exendin-9 (Ex-9). Notably, obestatin binding in 3T3-L1 preadipocytes and adipocytes was prevented by siRNA against GLP-1R [23]. In agreement with the previous findings in pancreatic β-cells [21], these results suggest specific obestatin interaction with GLP-1R in adipocytes. Interestingly, obestatin secretion in both 3T3-L1 and human SC and OM adipocytes was increased during differentiation [23], suggesting that obestatin may be a novel adipokine exerting autocrine/paracrine effects, in line with other studies [24].

In vivo, mice injected intraperitoneally with obestatin and fed a high-fat diet (HFD) showed reduced insulin resistance and increased insulin sensitivity [23]. Obestatin reduced plasma glucose and increased plasma and pancreatic insulin levels, suggesting insulinotropic effects. Indeed, treatment with obestatin, besides counteracting HFD-induced reduction of islet area, strongly stimulated glucose-induced insulin secretion in islets explanted from both low-fat diet (LFD)- and HFD-fed mice. Moreover, epididymal fat from obestatin-treated mice fed an HFD showed increased glucose uptake with respect to untreated animals, and reduced glycerol release (lipolysis), which was increased by HFD. In agreement with the in vitro data, obestatin treatment in vivo also reduced HFD-induced apoptosis in fat explants. Obestatin also counteracted the inhibitory effect of HFD on adiponectin secretion by increasing adiponectin levels in both epididymal and SC adipose tissue. Moreover, it reduced proinflammatory cytokine release in fat, muscle and liver of HFD-fed mice and counteracted HFD-induced reduction of Akt and AMPK phosphorylation in these tissues [23]. Therefore, together with the in vitro data, these results strongly suggest a positive role of obestatin in the regulation of glucose homeostasis.

Conclusions

It is becoming increasingly evident that the ghrelin system plays a key role in the regulation of metabolic processes, such as glucose and lipid metabolism. The complexity of the ghrelin system still has to be disentangled, due to the many unsolved questions, such as the identification of the receptor(s) for UAG and obestatin. AG behaves differently from UAG and obestatin on glucose metabolism, showing insulinostatic and diabetogenic effects. However, in pancreatic β-cells, all the ghrelin gene peptides display survival and antiapoptotic actions, indicating similar effects on cell survival and opposite exploitations in metabolism. Identification of the receptor(s) involved in these complicated outcomes would certainly help to clarify these conflicting findings. Moreover, the recent identification of GOAT had added further complexity to the system. Similar results have been obtained in adipocytes, although the actions of AG were found to be mostly similar to those of UAG and obestatin, particularly with regard to lipolysis or glucose uptake, and controversies still exist on these aspects. Unexpected interest has been recently addressed to obestatin, which was found to display a variety of effects in both β-cells and adipocytes. A positive role for obestatin in glucose metabolism has been suggested, as well as interaction with GLP-1R, which would at least partly explain its survival and insulinotropic actions, as well as its positive effects on insulin sensitivity in peripheral tissues. Additional studies are needed to understand the role of each peptide, their binding to one or more receptor and activation of signaling cascades in the different cell types.

Acknowledgement

This work has been supported by Compagnia di San Paolo (2008 to E.G. and 2011 to R.G.), PRIN 2008 to R.G., Brain Drain, University of Turin 2008, and SMEM Foundation, Turin, Italy.

References

1 Kojima M, Hosoda H, Date Y, Nakazato M, Matsuo H, Kangawa K: Ghrelin is a growth-hormone-releasing acylated peptide from stomach. Nature 1999;402: 656–660.
2 van der Lely AJ, Tschop M, Heiman ML, Ghigo E: Biological, physiological, pathophysiological, and pharmacological aspects of ghrelin. Endocr Rev 2004;25: 426–457.
3 Gutierrez JA, Solenberg PJ, Perkins DR, Willency JA, Knierman MD, Jin Z, Witcher DR, Luo S, Onyia JE, Hale JE: Ghrelin octanoylation mediated by an orphan lipid transferase. Proc Natl Acad Sci USA 2008; 105:6320–6325.
4 Yang J, Brown MS, Liang G, Grishin NV, Goldstein JL: Identification of the acyltransferase that octanoylates ghrelin, an appetite-stimulating peptide hormone. Cell 2008;132:387–396.
5 Sun Y, Wang P, Zheng H, Smith RG: Ghrelin stimulation of growth hormone release and appetite is mediated through the growth hormone secretagogue receptor. Proc Natl Acad Sci USA 2004;101:4679–4684.

6 Date Y, Nakazato M, Hashiguchi S, Dezaki K, Mondal MS, Hosoda H, Kojima M, Kangawa K, Arima T, Matsuo H, Yada T, Matsukura S: Ghrelin is present in pancreatic alpha-cells of humans and rats and stimulates insulin secretion. Diabetes 2002;51: 124–129.

7 Dezaki K, Hosoda H, Kakei M, Hashiguchi S, Watanabe M, Kangawa K, Yada T: Endogenous ghrelin in pancreatic islets restricts insulin release by attenuating Ca^{2+} signaling in beta-cells: implication in the glycemic control in rodents. Diabetes 2004;53:3142–3151.

8 Gnanapavan S, Kola B, Bustin SA, Morris DG, McGee P, Fairclough P, Bhattacharya S, Carpenter R, Grossman AB, Korbonits M: The tissue distribution of the mRNA of ghrelin and subtypes of its receptor, GHS-R, in humans. J Clin Endocrinol Metab 2002; 87:2988.

9 Kos K, Harte AL, O'Hare PJ, Kumar S, McTernan PG: Ghrelin and the differential regulation of desacyl (DSG) and oct-anoyl ghrelin (OTG) in human adipose tissue (AT). Clin Endocrinol (Oxf) 2009;70: 383–389.

10 Gurriaran-Rodriguez U, Al-Massadi O, Crujeiras AB, Mosteiro CS, Amil-Diz M, Beiroa D, Nogueiras R, Seoane LM, Gallego R, Pazos Y, Casanueva FF, Camina JP: Preproghrelin expression is a key target for insulin action on adipogenesis. J Endocrinol 2011; 210:R1–7.

11 Hosoda H, Kojima M, Mizushima T, Shimizu S, Kangawa K: Structural divergence of human ghrelin. Identification of multiple ghrelin-derived molecules produced by post-translational processing. J Biol Chem 2003;278:64–70.

12 Granata R, Settanni F, Biancone L, Trovato L, Nano R, Bertuzzi F, Destefanis S, Annunziata M, Martinetti M, Catapano F, Ghe C, Isgaard J, Papotti M, Ghigo E, Muccioli G: Acylated and unacylated ghrelin promote proliferation and inhibit apoptosis of pancreatic beta-cells and human islets: involvement of 3′,5′-cyclic adenosine monophosphate/protein kinase A, extracellular signal-regulated kinase 1/2, and phosphatidyl inositol 3-kinase/Akt signaling. Endocrinology 2007;148:512–529.

13 Muccioli G, Baragli A, Granata R, Papotti M, Ghigo E: Heterogeneity of ghrelin/growth hormone secretagogue receptors. Toward the understanding of the molecular identity of novel ghrelin/GHS receptors. Neuroendocrinology 2007;86:147–164.

14 Benso A, St-Pierre DH, Prodam F, Gramaglia E, Granata R, van der Lely AJ, Ghigo E, Broglio F: Metabolic effects of overnight continuous infusion of unacylated ghrelin in humans. Eur J Endocrinol 2012;166:911–916.

15 Baldanzi G, Filigheddu N, Cutrupi S, Catapano F, Bonissoni S, Fubini A, Malan D, Baj G, Granata R, Broglio F, Papotti M, Surico N, Bussolino F, Isgaard J, Deghenghi R, Sinigaglia F, Prat M, Muccioli G, Ghigo E, Graziani A: Ghrelin and des-acyl ghrelin inhibit cell death in cardiomyocytes and endothelial cells through ERK1/2 and PI 3-kinase/AKT. J Cell Biol 2002;159:1029–1037.

16 Zhang JV, Ren PG, Avsian-Kretchmer O, Luo CW, Rauch R, Klein C, Hsueh AJ: Obestatin, a peptide encoded by the ghrelin gene, opposes ghrelin's effects on food intake. Science 2005;310:996–999.

17 Zhang JV, Jahr H, Luo CW, Klein C, Van Kolen K, Ver Donck L, De A, Baart E, Li J, Moechars D, Hsueh AJ: Obestatin induction of early-response gene expression in gastrointestinal and adipose tissues and the mediatory role of G protein-coupled receptor, GPR39. Mol Endocrinol 2008;22:1464–1475.

18 Chartrel N, Alvear-Perez R, Leprince J, Iturrioz X, Reaux-Le Goazigo A, Audinot V, Chomarat P, Coge F, Nosjean O, Rodriguez M, Galizzi JP, Boutin JA, Vaudry H, Llorens-Cortes C: Comment on 'Obestatin, a peptide encoded by the ghrelin gene, opposes ghrelin's effects on food intake'. Science 2007;315:766; author reply 766.

19 Tremblay F, Perreault M, Klaman LD, Tobin JF, Smith E, Gimeno RE: Normal food intake and body weight in mice lacking the G protein-coupled receptor GPR39. Endocrinology 2007;148:501–506.

20 Gronberg M, Tsolakis AV, Magnusson L, Janson ET, Saras J: Distribution of obestatin and ghrelin in human tissues: immunoreactive cells in the gastrointestinal tract, pancreas, and mammary glands. J Histochem Cytochem 2008;56:793–801.

21 Granata R, Settanni F, Gallo D, Trovato L, Biancone L, Cantaluppi V, Nano R, Annunziata M, Campiglia P, Arnoletti E, Ghe C, Volante M, Papotti M, Muccioli G, Ghigo E: Obestatin promotes survival of pancreatic beta-cells and human islets and induces expression of genes involved in the regulation of beta-cell mass and function. Diabetes 2008;57:967–979.

22 Miegueu P, St Pierre D, Broglio F, Cianflone K: Effect of desacyl ghrelin, obestatin and related peptides on triglyceride storage, metabolism and GHSR signaling in 3T3-L1 adipocytes. J Cell Biochem 2011;112: 704–714.

23 Granata R, Gallo D, Luque RM, Baragli A, Scarlatti F, Grande C, Gesmundo I, Córdoba-Chacón J, Bergandi L, Settanni F, Togliatto G, Volante M, Garetto S, Annunziata M, Chanclón B, Gargantini E, Rocchietto S, Matera L, Datta G, Morino M, Brizzi MF, Ong H, Camussi G, Castaño JP, Papotti M, Ghigo E: Obestatin regulates adipocyte function and protects against diet-induced insulin resistance and inflammation. FASEB J 2012;26:3393–3411.

24 Gurriaran-Rodriguez U, Al-Massadi O, Roca-Rivada A, Crujeiras AB, Gallego R, Pardo M, Seoane LM, Pazos Y, Casanueva FF, Camina JP: Obestatin as a regulator of adipocyte metabolism and adipogenesis. J Cell Mol Med 2011;15:1927–1940.
25 Dezaki K, Sone H, Koizumi M, Nakata M, Kakei M, Nagai H, Hosoda H, Kangawa K, Yada T: Blockade of pancreatic islet-derived ghrelin enhances insulin secretion to prevent high-fat diet-induced glucose intolerance. Diabetes 2006;55:3486–3493.
26 Kageyama H, Funahashi H, Hirayama M, Takenoya F, Kita T, Kato S, Sakurai J, Lee EY, Inoue S, Date Y, Nakazato M, Kangawa K, Shioda S: Morphological analysis of ghrelin and its receptor distribution in the rat pancreas. Regul Pept 2005;126:67–71.
27 Chanoine JP, Wong AC: Ghrelin gene expression is markedly higher in fetal pancreas compared with fetal stomach: effect of maternal fasting. Endocrinology 2004;145:3813–3820.
28 Wierup N, Svensson H, Mulder H, Sundler F: The ghrelin cell: a novel developmentally regulated islet cell in the human pancreas. Regul Pept 2002;107:63–69.
29 Andralojc KM, Mercalli A, Nowak KW, Albarello L, Calcagno R, Luzi L, Bonifacio E, Doglioni C, Piemonti L: Ghrelin-producing epsilon cells in the developing and adult human pancreas. Diabetologia 2009;52:486–493.
30 Wierup N, Yang S, McEvilly RJ, Mulder H, Sundler F: Ghrelin is expressed in a novel endocrine cell type in developing rat islets and inhibits insulin secretion from INS-1 (832/13) cells. J Histochem Cytochem 2004;52:301–310.
31 Hill JT, Mastracci TL, Vinton C, Doyle ML, Anderson KR, Loomis ZL, Schrunk JM, Minic AD, Prabakar KR, Pugliese A, Sun Y, Smith RG, Sussel L: Ghrelin is dispensable for embryonic pancreatic islet development and differentiation. Regul Pept 2009;157:51–56.
32 Prado CL, Pugh-Bernard AE, Elghazi L, Sosa-Pineda B, Sussel L: Ghrelin cells replace insulin-producing beta cells in two mouse models of pancreas development. Proc Natl Acad Sci USA 2004;101:2924–2929.
33 Adeghate E, Ponery AS: Ghrelin stimulates insulin secretion from the pancreas of normal and diabetic rats. J Neuroendocrinol 2002;14:555–560.
34 Portela-Gomes GM, Johansson H, Olding L, Grimelius L: Co-localization of neuroendocrine hormones in the human fetal pancreas. Eur J Endocrinol 1999;141:526–533.
35 Vignjevic S, Todorovic V, Damjanovic S, Budec M, Mitrovic O, Djikic D, Drndarevic N, Micic M, Miskovic-Krivokapic J, Djuricic S, Nikolic I: Similar developmental patterns of ghrelin- and glucagon-expressing cells in the human pancreas. Cells Tissues Organs 2012.
36 Hasselby JP, Maroun LL, Federspiel BH, Vainer B: Ghrelin in the fetal pancreas – a digital quantitation study. APMIS 2012;120:157–166.
37 Walia P, Asadi A, Kieffer TJ, Johnson JD, Chanoine JP: Ontogeny of ghrelin, obestatin, preproghrelin, and prohormone convertases in rat pancreas and stomach. Pediatr Res 2009;65:39–44.
38 Granata R, Baragli A, Settanni F, Scarlatti F, Ghigo E: Unraveling the role of the ghrelin gene peptides in the endocrine pancreas. J Mol Endocrinol 2010;45:107–118.
39 Ueberberg B, Unger N, Saeger W, Mann K, Petersenn S: Expression of ghrelin and its receptor in human tissues. Horm Metab Res 2009;41:814–821.
40 Volante M, Rosas R, Ceppi P, Rapa I, Cassoni P, Wiedenmann B, Settanni F, Granata R, Papotti M: Obestatin in human neuroendocrine tissues and tumours: expression and effect on tumour growth. J Pathol 2009;218:458–466.
41 Zhao CM, Furnes MW, Stenstrom B, Kulseng B, Chen D: Characterization of obestatin- and ghrelin-producing cells in the gastrointestinal tract and pancreas of rats: an immunohistochemical and electron-microscopic study. Cell Tissue Res 2008;331:575–587.
42 Briggs DI, Andrews ZB: A recent update on the role of ghrelin in glucose homeostasis. Curr Diabetes Rev 2011;7:201–207.
43 Stengel A, Tache Y: Ghrelin – a pleiotropic hormone secreted from endocrine x/a-like cells of the stomach. Front Neurosci 2012;6:24.
44 Filigheddu N, Gnocchi VF, Coscia M, Cappelli M, Porporato PE, Taulli R, Traini S, Baldanzi G, Chianale F, Cutrupi S, Arnoletti E, Ghe C, Fubini A, Surico N, Sinigaglia F, Ponzetto C, Muccioli G, Crepaldi T, Graziani A: Ghrelin and des-acyl ghrelin promote differentiation and fusion of C2C12 skeletal muscle cells. Mol Biol Cell 2007;18:986–994.
45 Granata R, Settanni F, Trovato L, Destefanis S, Gallo D, Martinetti M, Ghigo E, Muccioli G: Unacylated as well as acylated ghrelin promotes cell survival and inhibit apoptosis in HIT-T15 pancreatic beta-cells. J Endocrinol Invest 2006;29:RC19–RC22.
46 Mandrup-Poulsen T: Beta-cell apoptosis: stimuli and signaling. Diabetes 2001;50(suppl 1):S58–S63.
47 Muccioli G, Pons N, Ghe C, Catapano F, Granata R, Ghigo E: Ghrelin and des-acyl ghrelin both inhibit isoproterenol-induced lipolysis in rat adipocytes via a non-type 1a growth hormone secretagogue receptor. Eur J Pharmacol 2004;498:27–35.
48 McCabe C, Samali A, O'Brien T: beta cell cytoprotective strategies: establishing the relative roles for iNOS and ROS. Biochem Biophys Res Commun 2006;342:1240–1248.

49 Zhang Y, Ying B, Shi L, Fan H, Yang D, Xu D, Wei Y, Hu X, Zhang Y, Zhang X, Wang T, Liu D, Dou L, Chen G, Jiang F, Wen F: Ghrelin inhibit cell apoptosis in pancreatic beta cell line HIT-T15 via mitogen-activated protein kinase/phosphoinositide 3-kinase pathways. Toxicology 2007;237:194–202.
50 Wang W, Liu Y, Chen Y, Cao C, Xiang Y, Zhang D, Han L, Zhao H, Liu G: Inhibition of Foxo1 mediates protective effects of ghrelin against lipotoxicity in MIN6 pancreatic beta-cells. Peptides 2010;31:307–314.
51 Wang W, Zhang D, Zhao H, Chen Y, Liu Y, Cao C, Han L, Liu G: Ghrelin inhibits cell apoptosis induced by lipotoxicity in pancreatic beta-cell line. Regul Pept 2010;161:43–50.
52 Granata R, Settanni F, Julien M, Nano R, Togliatto G, Trombetta A, Gallo D, Piemonti L, Brizzi MF, Abribat T, van Der Lely AJ, Ghigo E: Des-acyl ghrelin fragments and analogues promote survival of pancreatic beta-cells and human pancreatic islets and prevent diabetes in streptozotocin-treated rats. J Med Chem 2012;55:2585–2596.
53 Egido EM, Hernandez R, Marco J, Silvestre RA: Effect of obestatin on insulin, glucagon and somatostatin secretion in the perfused rat pancreas. Regul Pept 2008.
54 Tremblay F, Richard AM, Will S, Syed J, Stedman N, Perreault M, Gimeno RE: Disruption of G protein-coupled receptor 39 impairs insulin secretion in vivo. Endocrinology 2009;150:2586–2595.
55 Jhala US, Canettieri G, Screaton RA, Kulkarni RN, Krajewski S, Reed J, Walker J, Lin X, White M, Montminy M: cAMP promotes pancreatic beta-cell survival via CREB-mediated induction of IRS2. Genes Dev 2003;17:1575–1580.
56 Cheng H, Straub SG, Sharp GW: Inhibitory role of Src family tyrosine kinases on Ca2+-dependent insulin release. Am J Physiol Endocrinol Metab 2007;292:E845–E852.
57 Favaro E, Granata R, Miceli I, Baragli A, Settanni F, Cavallo Perin P, Ghigo E, Camussi G, Zanone MM: The ghrelin gene products and exendin-4 promote survival of human pancreatic islet endothelial cells in hyperglycaemic conditions, through phosphoinositide 3-kinase/Akt, extracellular signal-related kinase (ERK)1/2 and cAMP/protein kinase A (PKA) signalling pathways. Diabetologia 2012;55:1058–1070.
58 Irako T, Akamizu T, Hosoda H, Iwakura H, Ariyasu H, Tojo K, Tajima N, Kangawa K: Ghrelin prevents development of diabetes at adult age in streptozotocin-treated newborn rats. Diabetologia 2006;49:1264–1273.
59 Yamamoto H, Uchigata Y, Okamoto H: Streptozotocin and alloxan induce DNA strand breaks and poly(ADP-ribose) synthetase in pancreatic islets. Nature 1981;294:284–286.
60 Ceranowicz P, Warzecha Z, Dembinski A, Cieszkowski J, Dembinski M, Sendur R, Kusnierz-Cabala B, Tomaszewska R, Kuwahara A, Kato I: Pretreatment with obestatin inhibits the development of cerulein-induced pancreatitis. J Physiol Pharmacol 2009;60:95–101.
61 Warzecha Z, Ceranowicz P, Dembinski A, Cieszkowski J, Kusnierz-Cabala B, Tomaszewska R, Kuwahara A, Kato I: Therapeutic effect of ghrelin in the course of cerulein-induced acute pancreatitis in rats. J Physiol Pharmacol 2010;61:419–427.
62 Kerem M, Salman B, Ozsoy S, Pasaoglu H, Bedirli A, Haziroglu R, Yilmaz TU: Exogenous ghrelin enhances endocrine and exocrine regeneration in pancreatectomized rats. J Gastrointest Surg 2009;13:775–783.
63 Ahima RS, Flier JS: Adipose tissue as an endocrine organ. Trends Endocrinol Metab 2000;11:327–332.
64 Soares VM, Garcia-Souza EP, Lacerda-Miranda G, Moura AS: Early life overfeeding decreases acylated ghrelin circulating levels and upregulates GHSR1a signaling pathway in white adipose tissue of obese young mice. Regul Pept 2012;174:6–11.
65 Kim MS, Yoon CY, Jang PG, Park YJ, Shin CS, Park HS, Ryu JW, Pak YK, Park JY, Lee KU, Kim SY, Lee HK, Kim YB, Park KS: The mitogenic and antiapoptotic actions of ghrelin in 3T3-L1 adipocytes. Mol Endocrinol 2004;18:2291–2301.
66 Choi K, Roh SG, Hong YH, Shrestha YB, Hishikawa D, Chen C, Kojima M, Kangawa K, Sasaki S: The role of ghrelin and growth hormone secretagogues receptor on rat adipogenesis. Endocrinology 2003;144:754–759.
67 Patel AD, Stanley SA, Murphy KG, Frost GS, Gardiner JV, Kent AS, White NE, Ghatei MA, Bloom SR: Ghrelin stimulates insulin-induced glucose uptake in adipocytes. Regul Pept 2006;134:17–22.
68 Davies JS, Kotokorpi P, Eccles SR, Barnes SK, Tokarczuk PF, Allen SK, Whitworth HS, Guschina IA, Evans BA, Mode A, Zigman JM, Wells T: Ghrelin induces abdominal obesity via GHS-R-dependent lipid retention. Mol Endocrinol 2009;23:914–924.
69 Rodriguez A, Gomez-Ambrosi J, Catalan V, Gil MJ, Becerril S, Sainz N, Silva C, Salvador J, Colina I, Fruhbeck G: Acylated and desacyl ghrelin stimulate lipid accumulation in human visceral adipocytes. Int J Obes (Lond) 2009;33:541–552.
70 Fontenot E, DeVente JE, Seidel ER: Obestatin and ghrelin in obese and in pregnant women. Peptides 2007;28:1937–1944.
71 Zhang W, Zhao L, Lin TR, Chai B, Fan Y, Gantz I, Mulholland MW: Inhibition of adipogenesis by ghrelin. Mol Biol Cell 2004;15:2484–2491.
72 Tschop M, Smiley DL, Heiman ML: Ghrelin induces adiposity in rodents. Nature 2000;407:908–913.

73 Wren AM, Small CJ, Abbott CR, Dhillo WS, Seal LJ, Cohen MA, Batterham RL, Taheri S, Stanley SA, Ghatei MA, Bloom SR: Ghrelin causes hyperphagia and obesity in rats. Diabetes 2001;50:2540–2547.
74 Theander-Carrillo C, Wiedmer P, Cettour-Rose P, Nogueiras R, Perez-Tilve D, Pfluger P, Castaneda TR, Muzzin P, Schurmann A, Szanto I, Tschop MH, Rohner-Jeanrenaud F: Ghrelin action in the brain controls adipocyte metabolism. J Clin Invest 2006; 116:1983–1993.
75 Thompson NM, Gill DA, Davies R, Loveridge N, Houston PA, Robinson IC, Wells T: Ghrelin and des-octanoyl ghrelin promote adipogenesis directly in vivo by a mechanism independent of the type 1a growth hormone secretagogue receptor. Endocrinology 2004;145:234–242.
76 Perez-Tilve D, Heppner K, Kirchner H, Lockie SH, Woods SC, Smiley DL, Tschop M, Pfluger P: Ghrelin-induced adiposity is independent of orexigenic effects. FASEB J 2011;25:2814–2822.
77 Zhang W, Chai B, Li JY, Wang H: Mulholland MW: Effect of des-acyl ghrelin on adiposity and glucose metabolism. Endocrinology 2008;149:4710–4716.
78 Delhanty PJ, Sun Y, Visser JA, van Kerkwijk A, Huisman M, van Ijcken WF, Swagemakers S, Smith RG, Themmen AP, van der Lely AJ: Unacylated ghrelin rapidly modulates lipogenic and insulin signaling pathway gene expression in metabolically active tissues of GHSR deleted mice. PLoS ONE 2010;5:e11749
79 Tsubone T, Masaki T, Katsuragi I, Tanaka K, Kakuma T, Yoshimatsu H: Ghrelin regulates adiposity in white adipose tissue and UCP1 mRNA expression in brown adipose tissue in mice. Regul Pept 2005;130: 97–103.
80 Ott V, Fasshauer M, Dalski A, Meier B, Perwitz N, Klein HH, Tschop M, Klein J: Direct peripheral effects of ghrelin include suppression of adiponectin expression. Horm Metab Res 2002;34:640–645.
81 Mano-Otagiri A, Ohata H, Iwasaki-Sekino A, Nemoto T, Shibasaki T: Ghrelin suppresses noradrenaline release in the brown adipose tissue of rats. J Endocrinol 2009;201:341–349.
82 Giovambattista A, Piermaria J, Suescun MO, Calandra RS, Gaillard RC, Spinedi E: Direct effect of ghrelin on leptin production by cultured rat white adipocytes. Obesity (Silver Spring) 2006;14:19–27.
83 Lin L, Saha PK, Ma X, Henshaw IO, Shao L, Chang BH, Buras ED, Tong Q, Chan L, McGuinness OP, Sun Y: Ablation of ghrelin receptor reduces adiposity and improves insulin sensitivity during aging by regulating fat metabolism in white and brown adipose tissues. Aging Cell 2011;10:996–1010
84 Baragli A, Ghe C, Arnoletti E, Granata R, Ghigo E, Muccioli G: Acylated and unacylated ghrelin attenuate isoproterenol-induced lipolysis in isolated rat visceral adipocytes through activation of phosphoinositide 3-kinase gamma and phosphodiesterase 3B. Biochim Biophys Acta 2011;1811:386–396.
85 Vestergaard ET, Gormsen LC, Jessen N, Lund S, Hansen TK, Moller N, Jorgensen JO: Ghrelin infusion in humans induces acute insulin resistance and lipolysis independent of GH-signaling. Diabetes 2008;12:3205.
86 Yoshizaki T, Milne JC, Imamura T, Schenk S, Sonoda N, Babendure JL, Lu JC, Smith JJ, Jirousek MR, Olefsky JM: SIRT1 exerts anti-inflammatory effects and improves insulin sensitivity in adipocytes. Mol Cell Biol 2009;29:1363–1374.

Riccarda Granata, PhD
Department of Medical Sciences, University of Turin, Division of Endocrinology
Diabetology and Metabolism
Corso Dogliotti 14, IT–10126 Turin (Italy)
E-Mail riccarda.granata@unito.it

Benso A, Casanueva FF, Ghigo E, Granata A (eds): The Ghrelin System.
Endocr Dev. Basel, Karger, 2013, vol 25, pp 157–166 (DOI: 10.1159/000346065)

Clinical Perspectives for Ghrelin-Derived Therapeutic Products

Soraya Allas · Thierry Abribat

Alizé Pharma, Ecully, France

Abstract

Because of its orexigenic, adipogenic and diabetogenic activities, acylated ghrelin (AG) has emerged as an attractive target for the treatment of obesity and type 2 diabetes. Pharmacological tools have been designed in order to antagonize or block the hormone's activity, or inhibit ghrelin *O*-acyltransferase (GOAT), the enzyme that catalyzes its acylation. AG antagonists, shown to be potent inhibitors of growth hormone (GH) secretion, were not able to consistently induce the desirable metabolic effects. Some of them, on the contrary, acted as AG agonists. Similarly, AG-blocking agents including Spiegelmers, vaccines, and monoclonal antibodies, gave mixed results. More encouraging yet very preliminary data were obtained with a novel GOAT inhibitor. However, although significant, the observed decrease in circulating AG levels was partial and improvement work remains to be done. Unacylated ghrelin (UAG) and analogs were shown to potently and rapidly inhibit plasma AG levels, and to improve glucose metabolism in addition to displaying beneficial effects on a variety of cells. These data support the rationale for further development of this new therapeutic class in type 2 diabetes and the Prader-Willi syndrome. A development program is underway with AZP-531, a cyclized $UAG_{(6-13)}$ analog with improved pharmacokinetic properties.

The growing understanding of ghrelin biology has led to the identification of the ghrelin system as a pharmacological target for the treatment of a broad variety of diseases including GH deficiency, obesity, type 2 diabetes, gastrointestinal motility disorders and wasting syndromes. A couple of decades before the acylated form of the 28-amino acid peptide was identified as the endogenous ligand for GHS-R1a, orally available nonpeptidyl and peptidyl pharmacological compounds, the so-called GH secretagogues (GHS), were designed as potent stimulators of GH secretion. These drugs were initially developed with the hope of offering an appealing alternative to the daily subcutaneous hGH administration in childhood-onset GH deficiency and providing some benefits in normal aging. In the child, results of controlled trials have been globally disappointing as chronic administration of GHS produced modest acceleration of growth velocity. In the elderly, weight gain was noted because of the orexigenic and adipogenic effects observed in parallel to the increased lean body mass, and improvements in functional measures were inconsistent [1]. In addition, there was an increase in blood glucose. All of these unwanted effects clearly reversed the overall balance of benefits and risks for GHS in this type of clinical indication. Today, in both children and adults, GHS are considered for their potential use as provocative tests for the diagnostic of GH deficiency.

Effects of acylated ghrelin (AG) on appetite and body weight have subsequently provided the rationale for the development of AG agonists in the treatment of wasting syndromes and some large clinical studies are ongoing in cancer or chronic obstructive pulmonary disease cachexia with the challenge of demonstrating clinical benefits associated with weight gain. Also, based on stimulatory effects on gastrointestinal motility, the potential of synthetic small-molecule ghrelin agonists is being tested in diabetic gastroparesis and postoperative ileus. Although promising preclinical and clinical results were generated with TZP-101, a new intravenous administered agent [2], a recent phase 3 clinical trial assessing gastrointestinal recovery following partial bowel resection has failed to meet study endpoints.

On the other hand, antagonizing or blocking the effects of AG on food intake, body weight and glucose has emerged as an attractive target for the pharmacological treatment of obesity and type 2 diabetes. Globally, two approaches have been pursued and include generation of AG antagonists and blockers targeting GHS-R1a and AG, respectively, and GOAT inhibitors targeting the recently identified acyltransferase responsible for the ghrelin acylation. The positive correlation reported between circulating AG levels and insulin resistance has supported the effort in that direction. In parallel, experimental evidence has accumulated over the years with regards to the biological activities of unacylated ghrelin (UAG) through an unidentified receptor, distinct from GHS-R1a. In addition to improving postprandial glycemia, recent data indicate that administration of UAG significantly decreased plasma AG levels, in addition to its direct protective and regenerative effects on a variety of cells, positioning UAG and analogs as a promising way to treat type 2 diabetes and a third valuable approach to decrease AG in diseases and conditions where this could be beneficial. In this regard, clinical development program is underway with AZP-531, a cyclic analog of a UAG bioactive fragment with improved pharmacokinetic properties. This review describes and compares data obtained from the different pharmacological tools aiming at inhibiting or antagonizing effects of AG with the clinical perspective of getting desirable effects on food intake, body mass, and glucose homeostasis (fig. 1).

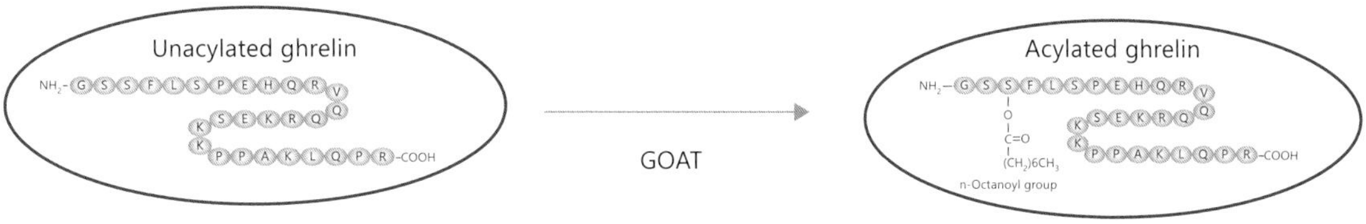

UAG agonists	GOAT inhibitors	AG antagonists and blockers
Animal and human data	Animal data	Animal and human data
Decrease in plasma AG	Decrease in plasma AG	Decrease in AG central activity as assessed by inhibition of GH secretion
Improvement in post-prandial glucose and insulin sensitivity Prevention of fat accumulation	Reduction in blood glucose and weight gain	Mixed results on food intake and body composition
Protective and/or regenerative effects on β-cells, EPCs and muscle cells	No data available	No data available

Fig. 1. Main effects of pharmacological tools aiming at blocking or inhibiting the effects of AG.

Acylated Ghrelin Antagonists and Blockers

GHS-R1a Antagonists

Academic groups and the pharmaceutical industry have been very active in this field and, as endocrine effects of AG on GH secretion were known to be mediated by GHS-R1a, classes of GHS-R1a antagonists were the very earliest drugs in this category that have been designed, using known or newly identified AG agonists and ligands. Modification of GHRP-6, the synthetic peptidyl GHS-R1a agonist discovered from early work by Bowers and coll, has resulted in D-[Lys3] GHRP-6, a selective antagonist able to decrease food intake in lean and obese rats [3]. Recently, the compound was shown to reduce body weight and glucose in a mouse model of postmenopausal obesity [4].

Piperidine-substituted quinazoline derivatives were identified as a new class of potent and selective orally bioavailable small molecule antagonists of GHS-R1a. YIL-781 and YIL-870, two of these compounds generated by the Bayer Research Center, were shown to block insulin secretion in vitro, decrease blood glucose after single dosing in lean and diet-induced obese (DIO) mice, and reduce body weight after daily dosing for 9 days in DIO mice [5]. Although plasma concentrations of the two compounds were comparable following repeat administration, brain levels were different. YIL-

870, which had a higher brain exposure, showed a greater decrease in body weight as compared to the other compound. Effect on body weight was due to selective loss of fat mass, was greater than the one observed with rimonabant, used as positive control, and accounted for reduced food intake. This latter effect was sustained for several days and did not recover at the end of the experiment to levels seen with controls. With YIL-781, brain concentrations were found to be 20% of plasma, and improvement in glucose homeostasis was better. Taken together, these observations have led to the hypothesis that the difference in efficacy and potency between the two compounds could relate to differences in central nervous system penetration, and therefore their ability to antagonize central versus peripheral acetyl ghrelin signaling system.

A series of potent ligands of GHS-R1a with a 1,2,4-triazole structure was discovered as in vivo antagonists of hexarelin-stimulated food intake. Administration of JMV2959 as daily subcutaneous injections for 2 weeks to DIO mice induced a reduction in weight gain and fat accumulation with no effect on lean mass. Interestingly, the reduced fat deposition was accompanied by reduced food efficiency, with no effect on food intake, suggesting stimulation of energy expenditure [6]. This antagonist has been recently shown to reduce alcohol intake in animals [7], suggesting therapeutic potential in alcohol use disorders.

BIM28163 is a peptoid analogue of full-length human ghrelin that has been developed by the Ipsen discovery group for its inability to stimulate h-GHS-1a receptor [8]. In vitro, when added in combination, BIM28163 completely and dose-dependently inhibited the ability of h-ghrelin to activate hGHS-R1a. In vivo, BIM28163 was observed to fully block ghrelin-induced GH secretion; the effect was specific to ghrelin as it was not seen when ghrelin was replaced with growth hormone-releasing hormone (GHRH). However, subsequent experiments showed that daily treatment with BIM28163 for 7 days had no effect on food intake and body weight in normal rats at a lower dose (40 nmol/kg) and, unexpectedly, induced an increase in both parameters at a higher dose (400 nmol/kg) to a comparable extent as that observed with h-ghrelin.

GSK1614343, a carbohydrazide derivative from the GSK laboratories, is a second example of potent and competitive GHS-R1a antagonist with regards to GH secretion that acts as an AG agonist for the feeding and body composition actions [9]. Increased food intake and body weight were observed following acute or chronic administration in two animal species, rat and dog. These findings were associated with increased both fat and lean mass (in the rat) and decreased both plasma AG and UAG levels (in the dog at the highest dose), suggesting that the compound directly or indirectly modulated both ghrelin forms in plasma.

Collectively, the observations from the Ipsen and GSK drugs have led to the hypothesis that the feeding and weight modulating actions of AG are mediated by an additional receptor that is distinct from GHS-R1a. Some evidence have been provided with BIM28163 studies comparing effects on two different hypothalamic areas, the medial arcuate nucleus (ARC) and the dorsal medial hypothalamus (DMH), known to be involved in the regulation of GH secretion and feeding, respectively.

Other GHS-R1a antagonists seem to be still under preclinical testing such as piperazine-bisamide analogs that were discovered as partial agonists and were converted to antagonists. However, published data to date indicate that no candidate of this class of drugs has moved into development.

GHS-R1a Inverse Agonists

Knowledge of the high degree of constitutive signaling activity of GHS-R1a has opened the way for the identification of inverse GHS-R1a agonists to inhibit appetite and food intake. In this attempt, [D-Arg^{1}, D-Phe^{5}, D-Trp^{7,9}, Leu^{11}]-substance P was identified to be a high efficacy and potency inverse agonist for GHS-R1a [10]. However, stimulatory effects of this agent of other receptors such as the substance P and the bombesin receptor may limit its use as a pharmacological tool.

The in vivo effects of GHS-R1a inverse agonists remain to be demonstrated but overall, GHS-R1a data suggest that the receptor may not be the appropriate target for anti-obesity and anti-feeding therapeutics.

Acylated Ghrelin-Blocking Agents

To date, blocking of AG has been investigated using Spiegelmers (synthetic polyethylene glycol-modified L-RNA oligonucleotide), vaccines and monoclonal antibodies. Spiegelmer NOX-B11, initially developed by Noxxon and subsequently by Pfizer and Merck, specifically attaches to AG, blocks its ability to bind to GHS-R1a and inactivates the hormone's stimulation of the receptor in cell culture. Intravenous administration of NOX-B11 to rats was shown to dose-dependently suppress AG induced release of GH and AG induced food intake, and to prevent AG's activation of neurones in the ARC of the hypothalamus [11]. NOX-B11–2, a second-generation anti-AG Spiegelmer, reduced food intake and promoted weight loss in a 7-day study in DIO mice; the effect was directly mediated by neutralization of AG as administration of NOX-B11–2 to ghrelin-deficient mice resulted in no weight loss [12]. Its successor, NOXX-B-11–3, is a long-lasting inhibitor of GH secretion that was observed to block AG but not fasting-induced neuronal activation in the hypothalamus ARC [13], suggesting that this agent may be efficacious in the presence of high plasma levels of AG. No further investigation of these Spiegelmer drugs has been reported and public information suggests that R&D programs have been discontinued.

High-affinity anti-AG-specific monoclonal antibodies have been recently generated and characterized. The lead compound of this series was shown to inhibit AG-induced calcium mobilization in vitro and AG-induced food intake following acute administration to normal mice [14]. No effect on food intake was seen when the drug was given after fasting-induced food intake following by refeeding. In the fast-refeeding challenge condition, the agent increased plasma AG while plasma UAG did not change, suggesting a compensatory mechanism that remains undetermined. Additionally, no effect on food intake and body weight was noted following repeat administration for 4 weeks in DIO mice although 99% of plasma AG was found to bind to the monoclonal antibody.

Therapeutic vaccine drug candidates were designed in order to induce production of specific anti-AG antibodies. Previous animal work showed that immunization with active vaccines based on the 28-amino acid sequence increased vaccine antibody titers with appropriate specificity after repeat administration [15]. Immunized animals gained less weight as compared to controls across the 7-day observation period after the last immunization, but no change in food intake was observed, suggesting a decrease in feed efficiency.

In the clinic, experience with therapeutic vaccine candidates has been however disappointing. A multicenter, randomized, double-blind, placebo-controlled trial involving 111 obese patients (BMI between 30 and 35) undertaken by Cytos Biotechnology AG showed no effect on weight loss, the primary endpoint of the study, and further development has since been stopped. In this study, patients received 4 injections of CYT009-GhrQb or placebo, and for those on the active drug, developed a strong antibody response against AG.

In summary, making Spiegelmers with high affinity to AG did not give the expected results, at least in the models that were investigated, and the global clinical potential of AG-blocking agents seems to be limited.

GOAT Inhibitors

GOAT catalyzes the addition of an octanoyl group on the serine in position 3 and is the unique enzyme responsible for ghrelin acylation. It is an intracellular enzyme, possibly located in the endoplasmic reticulum as acylation of ghrelin occurs before the preproghrelin hormone is translocated to the Golgi system where it is cleaved by prohormone convertase. Since the recent identification of the enzyme, its inhibition has quickly appeared as a potentially attractive target because ghrelin is the only known protein to be modified by acylation. Data have been recently published with regards to the design, synthesis, and characterization of GO-CoA-Tat, a peptide-based bisubstrate analog that antagonizes GOAT [16]. This compound was shown to inhibit production of AG, but not UAG, in two human cell lines that stably express GOAT, preproghrelin and produce both forms of ghrelin. In mice, serum levels of AG, but not of UAG, were diminished approximately by 50% following intraperitoneal administration of GO-CoA-Tat. In addition, chronic treatment for 4 weeks prevented body weight gain as compared to control. In this study, no evidence of generalized toxicity as a source of weight loss was reported, and blood glucose was lower in the treated group as compared to control. In an additional experiment, authors observed a reduction in weight gain in DIO mice associated with a reduction in fat mass while lean mass did not change. Interestingly, further investigation on glucose regulation showed that human islet cells exposed to GO-CoA-Tat induced a significant increase in insulin response to a glucose challenge. This effect was observed in wild type mice, but not in knockout animals, and was accompanied by a reduction in blood glucose.

Data obtained with GOAT inhibitors so far appear to be encouraging particularly when compared to findings resulting from investigation using Ghrelin antagonists. Much work remains to be done in order to optimize pharmacokinetic and pharmacodynamic properties, especially with regards to decrease in serum AG levels. Also, with GOAT inhibitors, the drug discovery work faces the challenge of designing compounds with cell penetration properties.

UAG and Analogs

Preclinical and clinical pharmacology results indicate that UAG, the most predominant form of circulating ghrelin, has non-GHS-R1a-mediated metabolic activities, sometimes supporting but most often opposing effects of AG. These data, extensively described in this book by Delhanty's group, have provided experimental evidence for the potential of UAG as an antidiabetic drug. Very early, UAG has been shown to display, in vitro and in animals, proliferative and protective effects on pancreatic β-cells; suggesting that UAG may prevent or delay loss of the endocrine pancreatic mass, an important target in the treatment of type 2 diabetes. In vitro, UAG as well as AG induced proliferation and inhibited apoptosis of two pancreatic β-cell lines, the HIT-T15 insulin-secreting cells (that express ghrelin but not GHS-R1a) and the INS-1E glucose-sensitive cells (that express GHS-R1a) [17]. In streptozotocin (STZ)-treated rats, UAG, similarly to AG, was able to reverse diabetes induced by STZ. In this animal model, UAG, differently from AG, increased the number of pancreatic islets and restored pancreatic islet area [18].

In order to identify the minimally active sequence of UAG, a series of analogs has been designed and screened for efficacy using the β-cell survival assay in both the INS-1E and HIT-T15 β-cell lines. Human islets obtained from pancreases of multiorgan donors were also used in these experiments. AZP-502, a linear 8-amino acid peptide (UAG_{6-13}) that does not include the serine 3 residue, the site for ghrelin acylation, appeared to be the smallest and most effective fragment of UAG in counteracting both cell death and apoptosis under either serum starved condition or cytokines [19]. In vivo, the peptide was shown to counteract the diabetogenic effects of STZ in rats as potently as the full length molecule.

As cyclization has been previously shown to increase the stability of small peptides, a cyclo-UAG_{6-13} analog has been designed (head to tail cyclisation) and named AZP-531. In the β-cell assay, the cyclic compound dose-dependently increased cell survival in both experimental conditions, similar to the linear form and UAG, their parent molecule. AZP-531 also increased glucose uptake from adipocytes and muscle cells similarly to UAG. In vivo, AZP-531 was shown to prevent weight gain induced by high fat diet (HFD), similarly to UAG, and to suppress fat mass gain [20]. These effects were observed with no change in food or energy intake. In this model, the compound, similarly to UAG, was noted to prevent HFD-induced insulin resistance. AZP-531 also prevented an HFD-induced increase in acyl ghrelin levels.

Plasma stability and pharmacokinetic properties of the linear and cyclic UAG_{6-13} analogs were investigated and compared [21]. AZP-531 has in vitro increased stability in human plasma; no degradation was observed even after 3 days of incubation while the linear form, subject to significant proteolytic cleavage, was degraded in its majority within 1 h and undetectable at 24 h. In animals, AZP-531, when given by the subcutaneous or intravenous route, was detected for up to 4 h (rat) and 8 h (dog) postadministration while AZP-502 was not present after 15 min (rat) and 30 min (dog) following dosing. In addition, mean subcutaneous bioavailibity was greater with AZP-531 versus AZP-502 (85 and 97% vs. 12 and 19% in rats and dogs, respectively).

A 15-hour infusion of 3 or 10 µg/kg/h UAG was shown to abolish plasma AG levels in a double-blind placebo-controlled study performed in type 2 diabetic patients [22]. At the highest dose, fasting AG levels were significantly correlated with the degree of decline in postprandial glucose concentrations. In the same patient population, a 75% reduction in plasma AG levels versus placebo was observed following a short-term infusion (2.5 h) of 10 µg/kg/h UAG. Collectively, these data indicate that UAG and AZP-531 may be potent inhibitors of plasma AG levels, explaining at least in part the observed metabolic effects, particularly the reduction of blood glucose. Plasma AG level may be a useful pharmacodynamic biomarker from a drug development perspective and a valuable tool for patient stratification and personalized medicine. Effects on AG levels also support the rationale for further investigation of UAG analogs in metabolic diseases or conditions where decreasing AG levels may be beneficial. A relevant clinical situation is given with the Prader-Willi syndrome, a rare endocrine hypothalamic disorder characterized by severe and compulsive hyperphagia leading to morbid obesity and for which no effective treatment is available. In Prader-Willi syndrome, plasma AG levels are markedly elevated, even prior to onset of obesity, and positively correlated with ratings of hunger.

In addition to its protective effects on β-cells and metabolic actions, UAG has been described to have protective effects on endothelial progenitor cells (EPC) and muscle cells. In type 2 diabetic patients, known to exhibit impaired EPC number and function, a 12-hour infusion of UAG, but not AG, protected EPC from senescence, increased cell mobilization and de novo vessel formation [23]. Both the linear and cyclic UAG_{6-13} analogs were also observed to prevent EPC senescence [19]. Initial in vitro work on cardiomyocytes showed that UAG, as well as AG, was able to inhibit cell apoptosis [24]. Additional investigation revealed the existence of a UAG-specific receptor in mouse cardiac cells [25]. Direct effects of UAG, as well as AG, was also demontrated on skeletal muscle cells including promotion of cell differentiation and fusion of C2C12 myotubes [26] and decreased muscle proteolysis following burn injury in rats [27]. Evidence was provided that C2C12 cells, which do not express GHSR-1a, contain a common high-affinity binding site recognized by both forms of ghrelin. Finally, very recent data suggest that UAG promote skeletal muscle protection and regeneration in a mouse model of hind-limb ischemia [unpubl. data]. Taken together, these findings suggest therapeutic potential in cardiovascular diseases, major complications of type 2 diabetes, including ischemia and reperfusion injuries.

Conclusion

Disappointing results have been obtained so far from the investigation of GHS-R1a antagonists, GHS-R1a inverse agonists and AG-blocking agents, and further testing has been stopped for most of these drug candidates. GOAT inhibitors could represent an interesting approach, and further potency with regards to AG inhibition remains to be demonstrated. Nevertheless, the long-term impact of suppression of some peripheral biological actions of AG, including protection of β-cells, remain questionable particularly when considering the type 2 diabetes clinical indication, and no published data is available. The use of UAG analogs may offer a novel and potent approach to improve glucose metabolism and inhibit AG levels while protecting cells and tissues, and may be of particular relevance to metabolic diseases such as type 2 diabetes and the Prader-Willi syndrome.

References

1 Merriam GR, Blackman M, Hoffman A, Salvatori R, Wei JY, White HK, et al: Effects of chronic treatment with an oral growth hormone (GH) secretagogue on nocturnal GH and insulin-like growth factor-I (IGF-I) in older men and women. Front Neuroendocrinol 2006;27:36–37.

2 Greenwood-Van MB, Kriegsman M, Nelson R: Ghrelin as a target for gastrointestinal motility disorders. Peptides 2011;32:2352–2356.

3 Beck B, Richy S, Stricker-Krongrad A: Feeding response to ghrelin agonist and antagonist in lean and obese Zucker rats. Life Sci 2004;76:473–478.

4 Maletinska L, Matyskova R, Maixnerova J, Sykora D, Pychova M, Spolcova A, et al: The Peptidic GHS-R antagonist [D-Lys(3)]GHRP-6 markedly improves adiposity and related metabolic abnormalities in a mouse model of postmenopausal obesity. Mol Cell Endocrinol 2011;343:55–62.

5 Esler WP, Rudolph J, Claus TH, Tang W, Barucci N, Brown SE, et al: Small-molecule ghrelin receptor antagonists improve glucose tolerance, suppress appetite, and promote weight loss. Endocrinology 2007; 148:5175–5185.

6 Roy MC, Paradis E, Samson P, Thiboutot-Gagnon N, Marcotte M, Lachance Y, et al: Long term treatment with non-peptide ghrelin receptor ligands affects energy balance in mice fed a high-fat diet. ENDO 2007:2–9.

7 Jerlhag E, Egecioglu E, Landgren S, Salome N, Heilig M, Moechars D, et al: Requirement of central ghrelin signaling for alcohol reward. Proc Natl Acad Sci USA 2009;106:11318–11323.

8 Halem HA, Taylor JE, Dong JZ, Shen Y, Datta R, Abizaid A, et al: Novel analogs of ghrelin: physiological and clinical implications. Eur J Endocrinol 2004; 151(suppl 1):S71–S75.

9 Costantini VJ, Vicentini E, Sabbatini FM, Valerio E, Lepore S, Tessari M, et al: GSK1614343, a novel ghrelin receptor antagonist, produces an unexpected increase of food intake and body weight in rodents and dogs. Neuroendocrinology 2011;94:158–168.

10 Holst B, Cygankiewicz A, Jensen TH, Ankersen M, Schwartz TW: High constitutive signaling of the ghrelin receptor – identification of a potent inverse agonist. Mol Endocrinol 2003;17:2201–2210.

11 Kobelt P, Helmling S, Stengel A, Wlotzka B, Andresen V, Klapp BF, et al: Anti-ghrelin Spiegelmer NOX-B11 inhibits neurostimulatory and orexigenic effects of peripheral ghrelin in rats. Gut 2006;55: 788–792.

12 Shearman LP, Wang SP, Helmling S, Stribling DS, Mazur P, Ge L, et al: Ghrelin neutralization by a ribonucleic acid-SPM ameliorates obesity in diet-induced obese mice. Endocrinology 2006;147:1517–1526.

13 Becskei C, Bilik KU, Klussmann S, Jarosch F, Lutz TA, Riediger T: The anti-ghrelin Spiegelmer NOX-B11–3 blocks ghrelin- but not fasting-induced neuronal activation in the hypothalamic arcuate nucleus. J Neuroendocrinol 2008;20:85–92.

14 Lu SC, Xu J, Chinookoswong N, Liu S, Steavenson S, Gegg C, et al: An acyl-ghrelin-specific neutralizing antibody inhibits the acute ghrelin-mediated orexigenic effects in mice. Mol Pharmacol 2009;75:901–907.

15 Zorrilla EP, Iwasaki S, Moss JA, Chang J, Otsuji J, Inoue K, et al: Vaccination against weight gain. Proc Natl Acad Sci USA 2006;103:13226–13231.

16 Barnett BP, Hwang Y, Taylor MS, Kirchner H, Pfluger PT, Bernard V, et al: Glucose and weight control in mice with a designed ghrelin *O*-acyltransferase inhibitor. Science 2010;330:1689–1692.

17 Granata R, Settanni F, Biancone L, Trovato L, Nano R, Bertuzzi F, et al: Acylated and unacylated ghrelin promote proliferation and inhibit apoptosis of pancreatic beta-cells and human islets: involvement of 3′,5′-cyclic adenosine monophosphate/protein kinase A, extracellular signal-regulated kinase 1/2, and phosphatidyl inositol 3-kinase/Akt signaling. Endocrinology 2007;148:512–529.

18 Granata R, Volante M, Settanni F, Gauna C, Ghe C, Annunziata M, et al: Unacylated ghrelin and obestatin increase islet cell mass and prevent diabetes in streptozotocin-treated newborn rats. J Mol Endocrinol 2010;45:9–17.

19 Granata R, Settanni F, Julien M, Nano R, Togliatto G, Trombetta A, et al: Unacylated ghrelin fragments and analogues promote survival of pancreatic beta-cells and human pancreatic islets and prevent diabetes in streptozotocin-treated rats. J Med Chem 2012; 55:2585–2596.

20 Delhanty PJ, Huisman M, Baldeon-Rojas LY, van den Berge I, Grefhorst A, Abribat T, Leenen PJ, Themmen AP, van der Lely AJ: Des-acyl ghrelin analogs prevent high-fat-dietinduced dysregulation of glucose homeostasis. FASEB J 2013;in press.

21 Julien M, Kay R, Delhanty P, Allas S, Granata R, Barton C, et al: In vitro and in vivo stability and pharmacokinetic profile of unacylated ghrelin (UAG) analogues. Eur J Pharm Sci 2012;47:625–635.

22 Özcan B, Neggers SJCMM, Miller AR, Yang H, Delhanty P, Allas S, et al: Rapidly and strong suppression of human acylated ghrelin serum concentrations during infusion of des-acyl ghrelin in obese diabetic subjects. Endocr Abstr 2012;29:711.

23 Togliatto G, Trombetta A, Dentelli P, Baragli A, Rosso A, Granata R, et al: Unacylated ghrelin rescues endothelial progenitor cell function in individuals with type 2 diabetes. Diabetes 2010;59:1016–1025.

24 Baldanzi G, Filigheddu N, Cutrupi S, Catapano F, Bonissoni S, Fubini A, et al: Ghrelin and des-acyl ghrelin inhibit cell death in cardiomyocytes and endothelial cells through ERK1/2 and PI 3-kinase/AKT. J Cell Biol 2002;159:1029–1037.

25 Lear PV, Iglesias MJ, Feijoo-Bandin S, Rodriguez-Penas D, Mosquera-Leal A, Garcia-Rua V, et al: Des-acyl ghrelin has specific binding sites and different metabolic effects from ghrelin in cardiomyocytes. Endocrinology 2010;151:3286–3298.

26 Filigheddu N, Gnocchi VF, Coscia M, Cappelli M, Porporato PE, Taulli R, et al: Ghrelin and des-acyl ghrelin promote differentiation and fusion of C2C12 skeletal muscle cells. Mol Biol Cell 2007;18:986–994.

27 Sheriff S, Kadeer N, Joshi R, Friend LA, Howard JJ, Balasubramaniam A: Des-acyl ghrelin exhibits pro-anabolic and anti-catabolic effects on C2C12 myotubes exposed to cytokines and reduces burn-induced muscle proteolysis in rats. Mol Cell Endocrinol 2012;351:286–295.

Soraya Allas
Alizé Pharma
15, chemin du Saquin, Bâtiment G
FR–69130 Ecully (France)
E-Mail allas@alz-pharma.com

Author Index

Subject Index